# Aging Gracefully

A Guide to Thriving in Your Nineties and Beyond

Donald West

Copyright © 2024

All Rights Reserved

ISBN: 979-8-9898682-7-8

# Dedication

Teenagers and youngsters have such an easy time coming to the Lord. This is especially true if their family attends church and does Bible study at summer camps. Fortunately, I fell into this category as my father attended a church called the Primitive Baptist Church, while my mother routinely visited the Missionary Baptist Church (better known as the Southern Baptist Church). My heart goes out to both, as they clearly saw the Word of God.

I came to know Jesus Christ as my Lord and Savior in late October at a Halloween party in 1942, soon after my tenth birthday celebration. The church program was about Halloween, but my heart was tuned to Jesus.

I thank my Lord and Savior, who is the lover of my soul, Jesus Christ, for inspiring me to author this book. This book is a part of the journey You allowed me to walk with You, and I am so grateful to You. It is because of You, my Lord, that I am where I am today.

Glory to You, and all honor to You for being in control of the wheel steering my life. It was Your goodness and mercy that guided and led me through my life journey of the last eighty-two years; I thank You for that. I dedicate this book to You because You are the Author, the Finisher of my faith, and the Keeper of my soul.

# Acknowledgment

I wish to acknowledge my Great Grandfather William Wiley West, now known as WWW, whom I visited in Lexington, Oklahoma, a few years before the one-hundredth anniversary of his birth, April 4, 1854. He was 99 years old at his death (July 31, 1953), having survived sunstroke at 93 while chopping cotton.

Even to this day, his extended family comes together in Purcell, Oklahoma, annually over the Labor Day weekend for the family reunion titled WWW in his honor.

It is believed that he served as a Drummer Boy at a tender age with the army of Arkansas and came to Oklahoma in 1912, accompanying his family after Oklahoma became a state.

Inspired by my Great-Grandfather's longevity, I am committed to healthy habits in hopes of living to 103 to see my granddaughter complete high school.

"Dear friends, do not let this one thing escape you;

with the Lord one day is like 1,000 years, and 1,000

years like one day.

--2 Peter 3:8

## Table of Contents

Dedication ............................................................................. iii

Acknowledgment ................................................................. iv

Preface .................................................................................. vii

Chapter 1: Embracing Change ............................................ 1

Chapter 2: Nourishing The Body ....................................... 16

Chapter 3: Mind-Body Connection ................................... 36

Chapter 4: Social Engagement ........................................... 55

Chapter 5: Preventive Health-Care .................................... 75

Chapter 6: Hobbies And Passions ...................................... 88

Chapter 7: Financial Wellness ............................................ 104

Chapter 8: Embracing Technology ..................................... 121

Chapter 9: Taking Charge Of Your Life ............................. 136

Chapter 10: Aging Like A Champion ................................. 150

About The Author ................................................................ 157

# Preface

As we stand at the crossroads of life, a new horizon stretches before us. The vibrancy of youth may be fading, but a different kind of strength emerges – the strength of experience, wisdom, and a life well-lived. Yet, the prospect of aging can be daunting. Images of frailty and decline might cloud our vision, leaving us unsure of how to navigate this exciting yet often-uncharted territory.

This book is for all those people who refuse to settle for a diminished existence. It is for those who yearn to embrace the coming years with vitality, purpose, and a healthy dose of swagger. Perhaps you see the first strands of silver in your hair, or maybe a creak in your knee reminds you that time marches on. Regardless, a powerful question lingers: How can we age gracefully, becoming the best versions of ourselves in this new chapter?

This journey is not about clinging desperately to youth. It is about embracing the unique gifts that come with age. We will delve into the often-overlooked psychology of aging, exploring how our perspectives and priorities shift. We will tackle the essential pillars of good health, both physical and mental, providing you with the tools to stay strong and sharp. But aging gracefully is not just about the body – it is about the mind and spirit as well. We will explore the power of purpose, reigniting that spark that fuels our passions and keeps us engaged with the world.

Through these pages, you will encounter strategies to redefine aging on your own terms. You will discover practical strategies for maintaining physical fitness, fostering mental acuity, and nurturing meaningful relationships. This book is not a collection of dry pronouncements – it is a conversation, a friendly guide on the path to becoming a distinguished gentleman.

So, my dear reader, turn the page and let us raise a glass (or a healthy beverage of your choice!) to the magnificent journey ahead and step into your best years yet. Get ready to embark on a journey of self-discovery and vibrant living. With a little planning, a positive attitude, and the wisdom you have acquired along the way, you can make the coming years the best part of your life!

# Chapter 1
# Embracing Change

Life is an ever-evolving journey marked by many transitions, and one of the most major transitions is the process of aging. As we journey through life, change becomes our constant companion. Every time, we see the world differently and learn new things, and yes, as we go through it all, our bodies change, too. Embracing change and gracefully aging means navigating these shifts with an open heart and a positive attitude.

Aging is an inevitable part of the human experience, encompassing a complex interplay of biological, psychological, and social changes. As individuals progress through life, they encounter a myriad of adjustments - physical, emotional, and cognitive. The psychology of aging delves into understanding how these changes impact our mental outlook and emphasizes the crucial role of cultivating a positive mindset to navigate this transformative journey with grace and resilience.

Imagine a garden where flowers bloom and seasons change. Each bloom has its own beauty, and the garden transforms as time passes. In the same way, our lives evolve with time. Our hair might turn a different color, our skin may show lines from countless smiles and experiences, and our bodies may feel different. Instead of fearing these changes, think of them as the blossoming of a beautiful flower in the garden of life.

Aging is not solely about chronological years; it is a multifaceted process that brings both challenges and opportunities. Physically, the body undergoes various changes, from decreased muscle mass to alterations in sensory perception. Psychologically, individuals may grapple with evolving identities, shifting priorities, and adjusting to new roles. These changes, if perceived negatively, can significantly affect mental well-being.

The theories surrounding aging shed light on the evolving priorities and emotional needs of individuals over time. Socioemotional Selectivity Theory suggests that as people age, they become more selective in their social interactions and focus on fulfilling emotionally meaningful goals. This shift underscores the importance of emotional satisfaction and positive experiences in the later stages of life.

## The Power of a Positive Mindset in Aging

A positive mindset plays a pivotal role in aging gracefully and maintaining overall well-being. As people grow older, embracing a positive attitude becomes increasingly essential in navigating the physical, mental, and emotional changes that come with aging. Those who adopt a positive mindset tend to experience reduced stress levels, better cardiovascular health, and improved immune function, contributing to a higher quality of life in their later years.

Cultivating a positive mindset is not just about maintaining a cheerful demeanor; it is a transformative approach to life that fosters resilience, adaptability, and personal growth. It involves embracing an optimistic outlook that acknowledges challenges yet chooses to approach them with a sense of hope and possibility.

Studies consistently show that individuals with a positive attitude toward aging tend to exhibit better physical health, greater longevity, and improved mental well-being. This mindset is not about denying the realities of aging but rather about embracing them with an attitude that seeks opportunities for growth and fulfillment.

Embracing a positive outlook on aging does not mean pretending everything is perfect. It is about accepting changes that come with getting older and finding ways to make the most of them. It is like seeing wrinkles as signs of a life well-lived instead of just signs of getting old. It is about staying active, being open to learning new things, and staying connected with others.

Also, aging gracefully is not about stopping time; it is about savoring every moment and finding beauty in each phase of life. Every experience, every wrinkle, and every change is a part of our unique story. The number of candles on our birthday cake does not matter when there is warmth and light, we carry within us.

Just like the garden that transforms with the seasons, we, too, transform as we age. Embracing change and aging gracefully is an adventure that includes finding joy in the small moments and being open to the surprises that life brings.

One of the key aspects of a positive mindset in aging is its influence on mental health. A positive attitude can mitigate the effects of common mental health issues such as anxiety and depression, promoting resilience and psychological well-being. This mindset shift often allows older adults to approach challenges with more adaptability and creativity, enabling them to find joy and satisfaction in various activities, hobbies, and social interactions.

Moreover, a positive outlook fosters a proactive approach to health and lifestyle choices. Older people with a positive mindset are more likely to engage in healthy behaviors such as regular exercise, balanced nutrition, and adequate sleep. This proactive stance toward health maintenance contributes significantly to their physical vitality, allowing them to remain active and independent for longer periods.

## Strategies for Cultivating a Positive Mindset in Aging

Here are the strategies that will help you age gracefully!

1. **Cultivating Resilience:** Developing resilience involves adapting to the changes of life and bouncing back from setbacks. Embracing change and learning from difficult experiences can contribute significantly to maintaining a positive outlook.

2. **Nurturing Social Connections:** Building and maintaining meaningful relationships play a pivotal role in fostering a positive mindset. Engaging in social activities, spending time with loved ones, and participating in community events can combat feelings of loneliness and isolation.

3. **Continuous Learning and Stimulation:** Keeping the mind active by pursuing new hobbies, learning new skills, or engaging in intellectual pursuits helps maintain cognitive health. It not only provides

mental stimulation but also instills a sense of accomplishment and purpose.

**4. Practicing Gratitude:** Cultivating an attitude of gratitude and being present at the moment can shift the focus from the negative aspects of aging to appreciating simple pleasures of life.

Aging is not a decline but an opportunity for personal growth, wisdom, and the cultivation of a resilient and optimistic mindset. Embracing this mindset will empower you to lead fulfilling and meaningful lives, transcending the challenges associated with aging and embracing the richness of the journey ahead.

"In all endeavors, if you are present, read what is available on the subject, and prepare, you will be successful and acquire the highest score (grade)." This timeless advice resonates profoundly when applied to the psychology of aging and the pursuit of a positive mindset. Being present in the moment is foundational to fully experiencing the nuances and beauty of transitions of life, especially the process of aging. It involves appreciating each moment, acknowledging feelings, and embracing the changes that come with growing older.

Staying informed about the psychology of aging through various sources is invaluable. Reading extensively on the subject, attending seminars or workshops, and seeking guidance from experts allow for a deeper understanding of the psychological intricacies involved in aging. This accumulation of knowledge equips people with a broader perspective, aiding in the development of strategies to foster a positive mindset.

Preparation plays an important role in shaping the outcomes of endeavors. Just as one meticulously prepares for a task or exam, the journey toward a positive mindset in aging requires deliberate planning, consistent effort, and the application of effective strategies.

By engaging in continuous self-reflection, understanding personal values, and setting realistic goals, you can proactively shape their mindset toward aging. This approach involves identifying potential challenges associated with aging, devising coping mechanisms, and embracing opportunities for growth and fulfillment.

The commitment to staying present, seeking knowledge, and preparing effectively serves as an important aspect in the journey toward embracing a positive mindset in aging. By internalizing these principles and consistently applying them, you cannot only enhance their mental well-being but also embrace the aging process as a transformative and fulfilling chapter of life.

## The Interplay Between Acceptance and Adaptation

Acceptance and adaptation are intertwined; they complement each other in fostering resilience and psychological well-being. Accepting the inevitability of aging facilitates the mental space needed to adapt effectively. Simultaneously, adaptation is fueled by the willingness to accept and embrace change rather than resist it.

Those who accept the aging process are better equipped to adapt to its challenges. They are more likely to seek help when needed, explore new opportunities, and find meaning in the different stages of life. This attitude of acceptance will enable you to approach aging with grace and dignity.

This acceptance of aging is not a passive surrender but an active engagement with transitions in life. It enables you to acknowledge the evolving nature of your circumstances and find innovative ways to navigate them. By acknowledging and understanding the natural progression of life, you can proactively take charge of your well-being.

Embracing the concept of aging as an integral part of the journey of life encourages a holistic approach to well-being. It helps people prioritize self-care, mental fortitude, and emotional resilience. This approach allows for a greater appreciation of the richness and depth that each phase of life brings, fostering a sense of fulfillment and contentment.

Remember, it is not resignation or passivity; rather, it is an active acknowledgment and embracing of reality as it unfolds. When applied to the process of aging, acceptance involves acknowledging and embracing the changes – physical, emotional, and social – that come with growing older. It is about making peace with the inevitability of aging and the wisdom it brings.

Resisting or denying the natural process of aging often leads to unnecessary stress, dissatisfaction, and emotional turmoil. Instead, accepting the inevitability of change allows individuals to redirect their energy toward adapting and finding joy and fulfillment in each phase of life.

## Strategies for Cultivating Acceptance and Adaptation

**1. Mindfulness Practice:** Embracing mindfulness cultivates an attitude of acceptance by focusing on the present moment without judgment. It helps individuals appreciate the beauty and richness of each phase of life.

**2. Flexibility in Thinking:** Encouraging open-mindedness and a willingness to explore new perspectives aids in adaptation. Embracing change rather than fearing it fosters resilience and personal growth.

**3. Seeking Support and Connection:** Building a strong support network and maintaining social connections promotes acceptance by providing emotional reinforcement and fostering adaptation through shared experiences and insights.

**4. Self-Reflection:** Engaging in regular self-reflection and practicing gratitude for the experiences and wisdom gained throughout life promotes both acceptance and adaptation. It encourages a positive outlook on the aging process.

As we progress through life, our definition of success also undergoes profound transformations, especially in the context of aging. The pursuit of success takes on new dimensions, shifting from traditional markers like career achievements or material gains to encompass broader aspects that focus on personal fulfillment, well-being, and meaningful connections.

In the earlier stages of life, success is frequently associated with accomplishments such as career advancements, financial stability, or acquiring possessions. However, as we age, our priorities shift, and the definition of success evolves. The emphasis gradually shifts from external validation to more intrinsic aspects that nurture emotional, social, and spiritual well-being.

Success in later years often involves finding fulfillment in relationships, maintaining good health, contributing to the community, pursuing hobbies, and deriving satisfaction from the simple pleasures of life. It is about feeling content, purposeful, and emotionally connected.

## Shifting Priorities in the Aging Process

As we grow older, we tend to rethink what truly matters in life. Instead of only chasing after accomplishments that others recognize, we start valuing feeling happy inside and cherishing each special moment. When our work duties decrease or alter, it gives us the chance to do things we love, like pursuing hobbies or spending time on activities that make us really happy.

Besides, as we age, relationships become super important. It is not just about what we do; it is about who we do it with. Building strong bonds with our family, friends, and the people around us becomes really valuable. Having these connections gives us a deep sense of meaning and happiness.

In this phase of life, many discover that doing things that bring personal joy and nurturing relationships brings a lot of fulfillments. It is like finding a new way of living where what makes us genuinely happy becomes more important than what others might think about our achievements.

Having more time to explore what we love can make us feel more content and satisfied. It is like getting the chance to rediscover ourselves and create a life that is more fulfilling and meaningful.

Furthermore, these connections we build and the moments we share with loved ones become the real treasures of our lives. It is not just about the things we accomplish but about the people we care about and the joy we experience together.

## Strategies for Redefining Success in Aging

**1. Adapt to Technology:** Start by familiarizing yourself with technology to stay connected with the world, as it opens up multiple new opportunities for learning and engagement.

**2. Celebrate Life Experiences:** Appreciate yourself even for the smallest milestones that you have achieved and the wisdom you gained through it. Recognize the fact that success can be measured in the richness of life experiences and relationships.

**3. Prioritize Connections:** Invest time in fostering and nurturing relationships that bring emotional fulfillment.

**4. Engage in Purposeful Activities:** Pursue hobbies, volunteer work, or activities that align with personal interests and values.

Redefining success in the later stages of life involves a profound shift in priorities, valuing personal fulfillment, connections, and overall well-being over traditional markers of achievement. By embracing this new definition, individuals can find deeper satisfaction, purpose, and contentment as they navigate the journey of aging.

Taking care of ourselves is crucial on this journey. Eating healthy, moving our bodies, and getting enough rest are like watering and tending to the garden of our well-being. It helps us feel strong and ready to embrace the new adventures that come with age. Keeping our minds active and curious, whether by reading new books, trying out puzzles, or learning new skills, adds colors to our garden of knowledge.

Remember, success is no longer solely measured by external accomplishments but by the richness of experiences, the depth of relationships, and the ability to find fulfillment and joy in every phase of life. Embracing this redefined notion of success paves the way for a more meaningful and rewarding life in the later years.

*"To every thing there is a season and a time to every purpose under the heaven"*

*- Ecclesiastes 3:1 KJV*

# Chapter 2
# Nourishing the Body

In the golden years of life, nutrition plays a crucial role in maintaining health and promoting longevity. Crafting a diet that caters to the unique needs of aging bodies is like planting the seeds of a vibrant and fulfilling life. In these later years, the body undergoes changes, and nutritional requirements evolve. Adequate nutrition is vital for seniors to support their overall health.

A well-balanced diet ensures that they receive essential vitamins, minerals, and nutrients necessary to keep their bodies functioning optimally. This can contribute to maintaining energy levels, preventing illnesses, and supporting various bodily functions. Let us explore the power of nutrition and unravel the secrets of a diet that can contribute to a longer, healthier journey.

As we age, it becomes increasingly important to adopt a nutritionally balanced diet to address the specific needs of the aging body. One significant change is the decline in muscle mass, a natural process known as sarcopenia. This reduction in muscle mass can lead to decreased strength and mobility, making it essential to focus on adequate protein intake. Including protein-rich foods, such as lean meats, fish, dairy, and plant-based sources, can help support muscle maintenance and overall physical function.

Metabolic changes also accompany the aging process, resulting in a gradual slowing down of the energy expenditure of the body. To counteract this, adjusting caloric intake and incorporating nutrient-dense foods, including a variety of fruits, vegetables, whole grains, and healthy fats, becomes crucial. Maintaining a healthy weight and preventing excessive weight gain can contribute to better overall health and reduce the risk of chronic conditions associated with aging, such as heart disease and diabetes.

Another aspect to consider is the alterations in nutrient absorption that may occur with age. Reduced absorption of certain vitamins and minerals, such as vitamin B12 and calcium, may necessitate dietary adjustments or supplementation. Regular medical check-ups can help identify any deficiencies and guide personalized nutritional recommendations.

Building a diet for longevity begins with a foundation of nutrient-rich foods. These include fruits, vegetables, whole grains, lean proteins, and healthy fats. These foods provide a diverse array of vitamins, minerals, antioxidants, and fiber essential for overall well-being. Let us discuss a few below:

### Fruits and Vegetables:

Packed with vitamins, minerals, and antioxidants, fruits and vegetables contribute to heart health, support the immune system, and help manage weight. Aim for a colorful variety to ensure you consume a broad spectrum of nutrients.

### Whole Grains:

Go for whole grains like brown rice, quinoa, and oats. These grains provide complex carbohydrates for sustained energy, fiber for digestive health, and various nutrients beneficial for aging bodies.

### Lean Proteins:

Include sources of lean protein, such as poultry, fish, beans, and legumes, to support muscle health and repair. Adequate protein intake becomes crucial as the ability of the body to build and maintain muscle diminishes with age.

### Healthy Fats:

Embrace sources of healthy fats, like avocados, nuts, and olive oil. These fats contribute to brain health, aid in nutrient absorption, and support joint function.

## Hydration: The Elixir of Life

Staying hydrated is fundamental for overall health, especially as we age. Aging bodies may be less sensitive to thirst, making it essential to consciously drink enough water. Staying well-hydrated supports various bodily functions and helps maintain overall health. Proper hydration supports digestion and joint health and helps maintain cognitive function. Aim for at least eight glasses of water a day and consider incorporating hydrating foods like water-rich fruits and vegetables.

Crafting a diet that aligns with the unique needs of seniors is not just about sustenance; it is a way to nurture and care for their well-being. It is an investment in a higher quality of life, allowing seniors to enjoy their golden years with vitality and fulfillment. By planting the seeds of proper nutrition, we contribute to a healthier and more resilient aging process, fostering a foundation for a fulfilling and vibrant life in the later years.

## Portion Control: Less is Sometimes More

Now, let us dive into the magic of moderation. Imagine your favorite treats – ice cream, pizza, or cookies. Now, think of enjoying them without overloading your plate. That is the beauty of moderation – finding the perfect balance between indulgence and keeping your tummy content.

When you manage your portions, you create a masterpiece. Not too much, not too little – just the right amount to satisfy your taste buds and keep your energy levels in check. Eating slowly in small portions might sound funny, but it is a game-changer. Imagine savoring every bite, letting the flavors dance on your taste buds. This slow approach gives your brain and stomach time to sync up so you know when you are full and can say, "Hey, that was just right!"

Your tummy has its own language, and it speaks through grumbles and gurgles. Through that, when it signals, "I am full," it is time to put down the fork. Avoid the temptation to stuff in that extra bite. Your body knows what it needs, and you just have to be able to hear it.

Stuffing yourself might seem like a good idea during a feast, but it can lead to discomfort later on. Your tummy works hard to digest what you eat, and overloading it can cause bloating, indigestion, and other not-so-fun feelings. Treat your stomach with kindness, and it will thank you later.

Eating is not just about filling your stomach; it is about appreciating the journey of flavors. When you practice mindful eating, you create a connection with your food. Take a moment to appreciate the colors, textures, and tastes – it is like a food adventure without the guilt.

Also, instead of mindlessly munching, choose snacks wisely. Portion out a handful of nuts or grab a piece of fruit. Smart snacking keeps your energy steady and prevents the crash that comes with overindulging in sugary treats.

Your body is your forever home, and treating it with respect is essential. Moderation in eating is like keeping your home tidy and well cared for. It ensures that your body functions smoothly, with just the right amount of energy and joy. Let us discuss a few strategies that will help you in controlling the portions.

**1. Plate Portion Control:** Use smaller plates to trick your mind into perceiving the food as larger portions. This helps in moderating your servings without feeling deprived.

**2. Hydration Habits:** Drink a glass of water before meals. This not only helps with hydration but can create a sense of fullness, making it easier to control portions.

3. **Listen to Hunger Cues:** Pay attention to your bodily signals of hunger and fullness. Eat when you are hungry, and stop when you are satisfied. It is about tuning into the natural cues of your body.

4. **Mindful Eating Practices:** Engage your senses during meals. Chew slowly, savor each bite, and appreciate the textures and flavors. This mindful approach helps prevent overeating.

5. **Plan Balanced Meals:** Include a mix of proteins, carbohydrates, and fats in your meals. This balance helps to provide sustained energy and can reduce cravings for excessive snacking.

Here is a pro tip - heart health is another priority for seniors, and a heart-healthy diet with balanced portions can contribute to longevity. This involves reducing saturated fats and sodium while increasing the intake of fruits, vegetables, whole grains, and lean proteins. Such dietary choices can support cardiovascular health and reduce the risk of heart-related issues.

## Staying Active is the Key

As important as it is to eat healthily, keeping your body active and healthy plays an equal role in nourishing the body. It is super important for seniors!

It helps your body stay strong, your mind to stay sharp, and improves your overall health.

With time, as the body ages, maintaining an active lifestyle becomes increasingly vital to counteract the effects of muscle and bone loss, joint stiffness, and decreased flexibility. Regular exercise has been linked to improved muscle strength, which is essential for maintaining balance and preventing falls—a common concern for older adults.

In addition to its physical benefits, staying active has a positive impact on cognitive function and mental health. Studies suggest that regular exercise can help reduce the risk of cognitive decline and may even contribute to the prevention of conditions like dementia. Physical activity stimulates the release of endorphins, promoting a sense of well-being and potentially alleviating symptoms of depression and anxiety commonly experienced in older age.

It is essential to note that the intensity and type of exercise should be tailored to individual abilities and health conditions. Consulting with healthcare professionals or fitness experts can help design a safe and effective exercise program that suits specific needs and goals. Here, let us explore some easy and fun exercises that you can do to stay active:

## 1. Walking for Wellness:

Walking is a fantastic exercise for seniors because it is easy on the joints, simple to do, and does not require any fancy gear. It is a low-impact activity that provides numerous health benefits. Aim for a minimum of 30 minutes of brisk walking on most days of the week – this could be a wonderful goal to work towards.

You do not need to find a special place for your walks; the beauty of walking is that you can do it almost anywhere. Take a stroll around your neighborhood and enjoy the fresh air and scenery. If going outside is not convenient, consider walking in a local park or even inside a shopping mall, especially if the weather is not cooperating. This flexibility makes it easier to incorporate walking into your routine.

Brisk walking means moving at a pace that gets your heart rate up a bit. It is not a race, so find a speed that feels comfortable yet slightly challenging. This kind of walking helps improve cardiovascular health, strengthens muscles, and can contribute to better overall well-being.

Aside from the physical benefits, walking can also be a social activity. Invite a friend or a family member to join you on your walks. It is a great way to catch up, share stories, and stay connected while engaging in a healthy habit.

## 2. Chair Exercises:

If walking feels a bit challenging, do not worry – there are seated exercises that can be just as effective. Find a comfortable chair, sit down, and get ready to move. Leg lifts are a great starting point; simply lift one leg at a time, then the other. This helps strengthen your leg muscles without putting stress on your joints.

For your upper body, try arm circles. Extend your arms to the sides and make circular motions. This helps improve flexibility in your shoulders and arms. If you want to add a bit of cardio, you can even march in place while sitting. Lift your knees up and down – it is a fantastic way to get your heart pumping without standing.

Chair exercises are wonderful because they provide support. If balance is a concern, you can perform these movements safely while seated. Always remember to sit in a sturdy chair, keep good posture, and move at a pace that feels comfortable for you.

Consistency is key, so aim to do these chair exercises regularly. You can start with a few minutes each day and gradually increase the duration as you feel more comfortable. If you have any health concerns or conditions, it is advisable to consult with your healthcare provider before starting a new exercise routine.

Chair exercises are a fantastic option for seniors who may have mobility challenges, providing an accessible way to stay active and maintain strength and flexibility.

### 3. Gentle Stretching:

Stretching is another wonderful practice that helps to keep your muscles flexible and can be adapted to your comfort level. Whether you prefer sitting or standing, gentle stretches focus on major muscle groups, promoting flexibility and reducing stiffness. These stretches can be incorporated into your daily routine and are especially beneficial for seniors.

When sitting, try simple stretches like reaching for your toes or gently rotating your ankles. If you are standing, you can stretch your arms overhead or do gentle side bends. These movements not only enhance flexibility but also improve circulation and joint mobility.

For a more structured approach, consider joining a yoga or Tai Chi class. These activities are designed to be gentle on the body while promoting flexibility, balance, and overall well-being. Yoga often involves various poses and stretches, while Tai Chi incorporates slow and flowing movements that engage different muscle groups.

Yoga and Tai Chi classes can also provide a social aspect, allowing you to connect with others while taking care of your health. Many classes are designed to accommodate various fitness levels, making them suitable for seniors with different abilities.

Remember to listen to your body and avoid pushing yourself too hard. Stretching should feel comfortable, not painful. If you have any concerns or health conditions, it is wise to consult with your healthcare provider before starting a new stretching routine.

Incorporating regular stretching, whether through simple at-home routines or organized classes like yoga or Tai Chi, contributes to maintaining flexibility, improving balance, and supporting overall physical well-being in seniors.

## 4. Water Aerobics:

Water aerobics is a fantastic option, especially if you enjoy spending time in the water. This form of exercise takes advantage of the buoyancy of water, which reduces the impact on your joints. It is a gentle yet effective way to stay active and healthy.

When you are in the water, your body becomes lighter, making movements more comfortable. Water also provides resistance, which helps tone muscles and improve overall strength. This is particularly beneficial for seniors, as it minimizes the risk of strain or injury that can occur with some land-based exercises.

Community pools often offer water aerobics classes specifically designed for seniors. These classes are led by instructors who tailor the exercises to accommodate various fitness levels and ensure a safe and enjoyable experience. Exercising in a group setting can also add a social element, creating a supportive and motivating environment.

If you are new to water aerobics, do not worry – classes are usually structured to be inclusive and beginner-friendly. You can start at your own pace and gradually increase the intensity as you become more comfortable. The refreshing feeling of being in the water makes the workout not only beneficial for your health but also enjoyable.

Before diving into water aerobics, it is advisable to check with your healthcare provider, especially if you have any existing health concerns. Once you get the green light, you can splash into a fun and invigorating exercise routine that supports your overall well-being.

## 5. Dancing for Joy:

Put on your favorite tunes and let the rhythm move you – dancing is a joyful way to stay active and have a good time. It is not just about exercise; it is also a fantastic way to express yourself and enjoy the music you love. Whether you are dancing in your living room, joining a local dance class, or trying out dance-based video games, there are many ways to incorporate dance into your routine.

Dancing is great for coordination and balance, two essential aspects of maintaining mobility, especially as we age. It engages various muscle groups, improving strength and flexibility. The best part? You do not need to be a professional dancer; just move your body in a way that feels good to you.

If you prefer a structured approach, consider joining a dance class in your community. Many classes cater to different levels, ensuring that everyone can participate and have a blast. If going out is not feasible, there are plenty of online resources and dance-based video games that make it easy to groove to the beat in the comfort of your home.

Dancing is a social activity as well. You can dance with friends and family or join group dance sessions. The social aspect adds an extra layer of enjoyment and provides an opportunity to connect with others who share your love for movement.

Remember, there is no right or wrong way to dance – it is about having fun and moving your body. So, turn up the volume, let loose, and dance your way to a healthier and happier you!

Pro tip - Do not forget that the most important part of any exercise routine is consistency. Make it a habit to include physical activity in your daily routine. Whether it is a morning walk, an afternoon stretch, or an evening dance, regular activity is the key to a healthier and happier life.

## The Essence of Quality Sleep for Seniors

In these years of life, the significance of quality sleep cannot be overstated. As we age, the importance of restorative rest becomes increasingly pivotal for maintaining overall health and well-being.

One of the primary factors influencing sleep in seniors is the natural evolution of the sleep cycle. As individuals age, they tend to experience changes in sleep patterns. Older adults often find themselves waking up more frequently during the night and experiencing lighter sleep. Understanding these shifts is crucial for addressing specific sleep-related challenges that seniors may encounter.

Quality sleep plays a pivotal role in maintaining physical health, especially for seniors. Adequate rest contributes to the ability of the body to repair and rejuvenate itself. It aids in muscle recovery, immune system function, and the regulation of various hormones. Seniors who prioritize quality sleep are more likely to experience improved cardiovascular health, reduced inflammation, and enhanced cognitive function.

Restorative sleep is closely tied to cognitive function, memory retention, and overall brain health. Seniors who consistently achieve quality sleep are better equipped to cope with daily challenges, process information, and maintain mental sharpness. In contrast, sleep deficiency has been linked to an increased risk of cognitive decline, Alzheimer's disease, and other neurodegenerative conditions.

The impact of sleep on emotional well-being is profound, and this holds true for seniors as well. Quality sleep is instrumental in regulating mood, reducing stress levels, and fostering emotional resilience. Seniors who prioritize restorative sleep are better equipped to navigate the emotional complexities that may arise during their later years, promoting a higher quality of life.

In order to enhance the quality of sleep for seniors, a multifaceted approach is often necessary. This includes creating a comfortable sleep environment, establishing a consistent sleep schedule, and adopting healthy sleep hygiene practices. Additionally, staying physically active, managing stress, and avoiding stimulants close to bedtime can contribute to a more restful sleep during the night.

Seniors may be more prone to certain sleep disorders, such as insomnia or sleep apnea. Recognizing the signs and symptoms of these conditions is crucial for timely intervention. Seeking professional guidance and exploring treatment options can significantly improve sleep quality and overall health.

Seniors who prioritize restorative rest are more likely to experience enhanced physical health, cognitive function, and emotional well-being. Recognizing the evolving sleep needs of older adults and implementing strategies to promote quality sleep can contribute to a more fulfilling and vibrant life in the later years.

The well-being of seniors is closely tied to the quality of their restorative rest. When older adults prioritize getting good sleep, it can have positive effects on their physical health, cognitive function, and emotional well-being. Quality sleep becomes increasingly important as people age, and understanding and addressing the evolving sleep needs of seniors can make a significant difference in their overall life satisfaction.

Enhanced physical health is one of the key benefits that seniors can enjoy with proper rest. Quality sleep contributes to better immune function, helping the body fight off illnesses. It also supports heart health and helps in managing conditions like diabetes. When seniors prioritize restorative rest, they are giving their bodies the opportunity to heal and regenerate, promoting overall physical well-being.

Cognitive function, which includes things like memory and decision-making, is also positively influenced by good sleep. Seniors who make an effort to get quality rest are more likely to experience better concentration and mental sharpness. This, in turn, can contribute to a more independent and fulfilling life as they age.

Recognizing the evolving sleep needs of older adults involves understanding that they may require

*"3 He healeth the broken in heart, and bindeth up their wounds. 4 He telleth the number of the stars; he calleth them all by their names. 5 Great is our Lord, and of great power: his understanding is infinite. 6 The Lord lifteth up the meek: he casteth the wicked down to the ground."*

*- Psalms 147:3-6 KJV*

# Chapter 3
# Mind-Body Connection

As the golden years unfold, maintaining cognitive fitness becomes a priority for seniors seeking to lead vibrant and fulfilling lives. This is particularly important because cognitive decline is a natural part of aging; however, actively exercising the brain can slow down this process.

The mind, like any other part of the body, requires regular exercise to stay sharp and agile. First and foremost, a sharp and agile mind allows one to maintain independence. Being able to make sound decisions, solve problems, and navigate daily tasks independently fosters a sense of autonomy, boosting confidence and overall well-being.

Cognitive health is closely linked to emotional well-being. Seniors with intact cognitive function are better equipped to manage stress, adapt to changes, and maintain positive relationships. Hence, a healthy mind contributes to a more optimistic outlook on life, enhancing the overall quality of your golden years.

Maintaining cognitive fitness is also essential for preventing cognitive decline and neurodegenerative conditions such as dementia and Alzheimer's disease. Engaging in activities that challenge the brain can help build cognitive reserves, acting as a protective factor against age-related cognitive decline.

Your mind facilitates continued learning and personal growth. Whether it is picking up a new hobby, learning a language, or exploring technology, cognitive fitness enables seniors to stay curious and engaged with the world around them. This continuous intellectual stimulation promotes a sense of purpose and fulfillment.

Fortunately, promoting cognitive well-being does not have to be a daunting task. Let us explore a range of accessible and enjoyable exercises tailored specifically for seniors. From mental stimulation to mindful practices, these activities aim to keep the brain active, resilient, and ready for the adventures that each day may bring.

## Understanding Cognitive Fitness

Cognitive fitness refers to the overall health and functionality of the mental cognitive processes, including memory, attention, and problem-solving skills. As we age, it is natural for cognitive functions to undergo changes, but proactive efforts can significantly influence the trajectory of cognitive well-being. Engaging in activities that challenge and stimulate the brain contributes to the creation of new neural pathways, fostering resilience and adaptability in the face of aging.

To nurture cognitive fitness, it is essential to adopt a holistic approach that encompasses various aspects of well-being. Mental stimulation, social interaction, physical exercise, and a nutritious diet collectively contribute to maintaining a sharp mind.

It is not just about maintaining existing abilities but also about embracing lifelong learning. The brain has an incredible capacity for adaptation and growth, regardless of age. By engaging in new activities, acquiring fresh knowledge, and staying curious, seniors can walk on a journey of continuous learning that not only enhances cognitive function but also brings joy and a sense of accomplishment.

Maintaining a sharp mind is crucial for seniors to lead fulfilling lives. Cognitive fitness, or the ability to think, learn, and remember, can be nurtured through a variety of exercises. As seniors embark on this journey, it is essential to approach cognitive fitness with a positive mindset. Embracing new challenges, learning new skills, and staying curious can contribute to a vibrant and fulfilling life during the golden years. Overall, a holistic approach that combines mental, social, and physical well-being is key to preserving cognitive fitness and enjoying a rich and satisfying lifestyle.

Let us explore some simple yet effective ways for seniors to keep their minds active and engaged.

## 1. Mental Stimulation: Sharpen Your Mind with Engaging Activities!

Engaging in mentally stimulating activities is like a workout for the brain. Reading books, solving puzzles, or playing strategy games can help keep the mind sharp. Consider joining a book club or participating in a weekly crossword puzzle challenge to add variety.

## 2. Social Interaction: The Key to Cognitive Wellness and Vibrant Living!

Staying socially active is vital for cognitive well-being. Regular conversations with friends and family, or even joining clubs or classes, can provide mental stimulation. Sharing experiences and ideas fosters brain health by keeping cognitive processes in motion.

## 3. Forever Learning: Discover the Joy of New Hobbies for a Thriving Brain!

Embrace the joy of learning by picking up a new hobby or skill. Whether it is painting, playing a musical instrument, or trying a new language, the brain benefits from the challenge of acquiring fresh knowledge. This not only stimulates the mind but also adds excitement to daily life.

### 4. Move to Improve: Elevate Your Mind with the Power of Physical Exercise!

Physical health and mental well-being go hand in hand. Regular exercise increases blood flow to the brain, promoting the growth of new neurons. Simple activities like walking, gardening, or even chair exercises can contribute significantly to cognitive fitness.

### 5. Mindful Moments: Meditation Magic for Stress Relief and Clarity!

Practicing mindfulness and meditation can help seniors manage stress and improve cognitive function. Techniques such as deep breathing, guided meditation, or mindful walking provide a mental reset, promoting clarity and focus.

### 6. Brain Buffet: Fueling Cognitive Health with Nutrient-Rich Foods!

A well-balanced diet is crucial for cognitive health. Incorporate foods rich in antioxidants, omega-3 fatty acids, and vitamins. Blueberries, nuts, fish, and leafy greens are known to support brain function.

## 7. Memory Mastery: Fun and Games to Keep Your Mind Agile and Strong!

Memory is like a muscle; it needs regular exercise to stay strong. Playing memory games like "Simon Says" or recalling a list of items from memory is a helpful activity. These activities challenge and strengthen the ability of the brain to remember.

Apart from this, keep in mind that staying organized is super important. You can do this by using calendars, to-do lists, and reminders for your daily tasks. This helps you feel less stressed and allows your brain to focus on important stuff. Another big thing is getting enough good sleep. Make sure you have a consistent sleep routine and a comfy environment for rest. Quality sleep helps your memory and keeps your mind clear.

Lastly, having a positive mindset is a big boost for your brain. Be around happy people, practice being thankful, and stay in the present moment. Being positive makes your mind healthier and helps you feel good overall. Doing these things every day can really make your mind strong and sharp, especially for older folks. It is never too late to take care of your mind!

Incorporating these exercises into daily life can significantly enhance cognitive fitness for seniors, promoting mental agility, memory retention, and a fulfilling, active lifestyle. Remember, it is never too late to invest in the health of your mind.

Simple exercises like puzzles, crosswords, and Sudoku can be enjoyable and effective in keeping the mind active. Regular reading is another beneficial habit, as it not only provides mental stimulation but also allows individuals to explore new ideas and perspectives.

Moving forward, let us dive into the world of reading and how beneficial it is for seniors.

## Nourishing the Habit of Reading – A Lifelong Adventure

The habit of reading is a timeless and enriching idea that transcends age, providing a gateway to new worlds, ideas, and perspectives. Embracing the joy of reading not only nurtures cognitive fitness but also offers a delightful escape into the realms of imagination and knowledge.

Encouraging seniors to make reading a habit can bring lots of good things to their minds. Reading is like giving your brain a workout, and it can be really enjoyable, too! Firstly, reading keeps the mind active and engaged. It is like taking your brain to the gym. When seniors read regularly, it helps them stay mentally sharp, boosting their cognitive abilities. It is a fun exercise that keeps the brain strong and healthy.

Secondly, reading can be a great way for seniors to relax and unwind. It takes you on an adventure without leaving your chair! Whether it is a fascinating story or learning something new, reading provides a break from daily worries. This relaxation can be especially important for seniors, promoting a sense of calm and reducing stress.

Moreover, reading can be a fantastic way to stay connected with the world. You get to have conversations with different characters or learn about different places and times. This connection is essential for mental well-being, preventing feelings of isolation and keeping the mind active and curious, like having a library full of knowledge at your fingertips. Seniors can explore new ideas, learn about different cultures, and expand their horizons through books. This continuous learning is not only enjoyable but also beneficial for maintaining a curious and open mind.

## The Benefits of Reading:

Below are a few benefits of reading:

**1. Cognitive Stimulation:** Reading is a workout for the brain, requiring mental processes such as comprehension, analysis, and visualization. Regular reading stimulates neural pathways, promoting cognitive health and keeping the mind agile.

**2. Stress Reduction:** Immersing oneself in a good book can be a powerful stress reliever. The act of reading transports individuals to different worlds, offering a temporary escape from daily pressures and fostering relaxation.

**3. Knowledge Expansion:** Books are treasure troves of information. Whether it is delving into history, exploring scientific discoveries, or understanding different cultures, reading broadens your knowledge base and fosters a lifelong love of learning.

**4. Improved Vocabulary:** Reading exposes individuals to a diverse range of words and expressions. Over time, this exposure contributes to an enriched vocabulary, enhancing communication skills and cognitive abilities.

**5. Enhanced Empathy:** Fictional stories and narratives provide insights into the lives and emotions of diverse characters. This empathetic connection cultivated through reading can enhance social understanding and emotional intelligence.

Pro Tip - Start small and gradually increase reading time. Set achievable goals, like reading a chapter a day, to make reading a manageable and enjoyable part of your routine.

Then, designate a cozy corner or chair where you can immerse yourself in a book without distractions. Ensure good lighting and comfortable seating to enhance the reading experience.

## Recommended Genres for Seniors:

Here are a few recommended genres for seniors that will help you choose your desired genre:

**1. Historical Fiction:** Transport yourself to different eras and learn about historical events through captivating narratives.

**2. Memoirs and Biographies:** Explore the lives and experiences of notable individuals, gaining insights into different perspectives.

**3. Mystery and Thriller:** Engage your mind with suspenseful plots and intriguing mysteries that keep you hooked till the last page.

**4. Inspirational Literature:** Read uplifting stories and motivational literature that inspire a positive outlook on life.

Nourishing the habit of reading is a gift you give to yourself—a journey filled with intellectual growth, emotional enrichment, and sheer enjoyment. As you embark on this lifelong adventure, remember that every page turned is an opportunity for discovery, imagination, and connection. So, open a book, lose yourself in its pages, and let the magic of reading unfold.

## Stress Management for a Peaceful Existence

In the hustle and bustle of life, stress can often become a constant companion. Identifying the sources of stress is the first step in managing it. Whether it is a specific situation, a recurring thought, or external pressure, understanding what triggers stress empowers individuals to address it more effectively.

Stress can manifest in both physical and mental symptoms, including muscle tension, fatigue, anxiety, and changes in mood. Being aware of these manifestations helps in adopting targeted stress management techniques.

It can be like a heavy load on our shoulders, but finding ways to deal with it is like giving our minds a helping hand. When we are stressed, our minds work over time, and we feel overwhelmed. Finding ways to manage stress, like taking deep breaths or going for a short walk, can be like pressing the reset button for our minds. It helps us feel more in control and ready to face whatever comes our way.

Stress can also affect our physical health, especially for seniors. It is like a sneaky troublemaker that can cause problems like high blood pressure or trouble sleeping. But when we manage stress well, we put a shield around our bodies. This can lead to better overall health, making sure our bodies and minds work together like a well-oiled machine.

Stress management is a secret weapon against feeling lonely or sad. As we age, things might change, and it can sometimes be challenging. But finding ways to cope with stress, talking to a friend, or doing activities we enjoy, for instance, is like building a shield against those tough feelings. It helps us stay positive and enjoy each day, creating a path to a happier and more fulfilling life.

Unfortunately, stress can even massively affect our memory and thinking. It acts as a fog that can make things a bit fuzzy up there. However, by managing stress through techniques like relaxation exercises or hobbies we love, we can clear away that fog. This can keep our minds sharp and focused, allowing us to enjoy the things we love doing even more.

## Stress Management Techniques:

For seniors aiming to lead a peaceful existence, effective stress management techniques are essential. Here are a few below:

**1. Mindful Breathing:** Practice deep, intentional breathing to calm the nervous system. Inhale slowly, hold for a moment, and exhale gradually. This simple technique can be done anywhere, providing instant relief.

**2. Relaxation Exercises:** Engage in relaxation exercises such as progressive muscle relaxation. Starting from your toes and working your way up, tense and then release each muscle group, promoting overall physical and mental relaxation.

**3. Nature Walks:** Connecting with nature has a profound calming effect. Take leisurely walks in a nearby park, garden, or nature reserve. The sights, sounds, and fresh air contribute to a sense of peace.

**4. Engage in Hobbies:** Immersing yourself in enjoyable activities like gardening, painting, or listening to music can divert your mind from stressors and provide a therapeutic outlet for creativity.

**5. Social Connection:** Maintaining social connections is crucial for emotional well-being.

Spend time with friends and family, share your feelings, and enjoy the support network that relationships provide.

**6. Time Management:** Organize your time effectively to avoid feeling overwhelmed. Prioritize tasks, break them into smaller, manageable steps, and give yourself breaks to avoid burnout.

**7. Guided Imagery:** Envisioning peaceful scenes through guided imagery can transport your mind to a calmer state. Picture serene landscapes or imagine achieving personal goals to reduce stress.

**8. Laughter Therapy**: Laughter truly is a medicine for the soul. Watch a funny movie, attend a comedy show, or engage in activities that bring genuine laughter. It releases endorphins, which are the natural stress relievers of the body.

Pro tip - Take a moment each day to reflect on things you are grateful for. This simple practice fosters a positive mindset and helps shift focus away from stressors.

Then, acknowledge that some things are beyond your control. Practice acceptance of the present moment, allowing room for emotional resilience and a more peaceful outlook.

## Emotional Well-Being: Nurturing Mental Health as You Age

As we navigate the various seasons of life, nurturing emotional well-being becomes increasingly important. From embracing healthy thoughts to cultivating positive relationships, the journey toward emotional well-being is an ongoing process that contributes to a fulfilling and joyful existence. Let us delve into the realm of emotional well-being, where the power of positive thoughts and meaningful connections holds the key to a mentally thriving senior phase of life.

Just as physical health is crucial, so is mental health. Emotional well-being encompasses how we feel, think, and cope with life challenges. Prioritizing mental health contributes to a more balanced and gratifying life.

Positive thoughts act as a beacon of light, guiding us through the ups and downs of life. Embracing optimism and cultivating a positive mindset can significantly impact emotional well-being.

### Nurturing Positive Thoughts

Here is how you can nurture positive thoughts:

1. **Practice Self-Compassion:** Be kind to yourself. Embrace imperfections and treat yourself with the

same compassion you offer to others. Acknowledge achievements and celebrate small victories.

**2. Gratitude Journaling:** Keep a gratitude journal to record things you are thankful for each day. Reflecting on positive aspects of life fosters a sense of contentment and elevates overall well-being.

**3. Surround Yourself with Positivity:** Cultivate a positive environment by engaging with uplifting people, activities, and content. Choose to focus on what brings joy and inspiration into your life.

Remember that building strong connections with family and friends is equally important. Make sure to talk and spend time together to feel like you belong and get emotional support.

Expressing your feelings is crucial for your emotional well-being. Talk to others, write in a journal, or find creative ways to express yourself. It helps you understand and deal with your emotions in a healthy way.

Change is something that happens to everyone. Instead of being scared of it, try to see it as a normal part of the life journey. Having a positive mindset about change can make it easier to handle.

Do not be afraid to meet new people! Try joining clubs or classes where you can meet others who share your interests. It is a great way to make new friends and have fun experiences together.

Pro Tip - If you ever feel overwhelmed by life changes, reach out for support. Talk to your friends, family, or even professionals who can give you helpful advice and coping strategies. Remember, you do not have to go through tough times alone!

Emotional well-being is a precious aspect of a fulfilling life, and as we age, nurturing our mental health becomes even more vital. By entertaining healthy, positive thoughts and fostering meaningful connections, seniors can navigate the complexities of life with resilience and joy. Remember, each day is an opportunity to embrace positivity, cultivate emotional well-being, and savor the richness that comes with a well-nurtured mind and heart.

So, taking care of our minds and bodies as we get older is like giving ourselves a special gift. We have learned that keeping our brains active through activities like reading, puzzles, and learning new things is crucial. Staying connected with friends and family, taking care of our physical health, and managing stress are like magic tricks for a happy and fulfilling life.

It is never too late to start taking care of your mind. Simple exercises, like reading a chapter a day or doing puzzles, can make a big difference. And do not forget the power of positive thoughts and emotional well-being – surrounding yourself with joy and meaningful connections fills your life with sunshine.

As we journey through the golden years, let us embrace the adventure of continuous learning, laughter, and taking care of ourselves. By doing these things, we can make every day special, full of discovery, and create a path to a happy and fulfilling life. Cheers to a well-nurtured mind and heart!

# DONALD WEST

*"Behold, I will bring it health and cure, and I will cure them, and will reveal unto them the abundance of peace and truth."*

*- Jeremiah 33:6 KJV*

# Chapter 4
# Social Engagement

In this chapter, let us dive into the wonderful world of building and maintaining relationships as we age. Just because the years are adding up does not mean our social lives have to slow down! In fact, nurturing connections with others becomes even more vital as we journey through the adventures of life. So, let us roll up our sleeves and explore how to cultivate meaningful relationships and promote social engagement that stands the test of time.

First off, let us talk about why relationships matter so much, especially as we age. Studies have shown that staying socially connected can boost our overall well-being and even extend our lifespan. From reducing stress to increasing feelings of happiness, maintaining strong connections with friends, family, and community members is like giving our hearts a warm hug.

As we age, it is natural for our social circles to evolve. Friends may move away, family dynamics might shift, and our interests could change. But fear not! Embrace the opportunity to meet new people and explore different social activities. Whether it is joining a book club, volunteering at a local charity, or taking up a new hobby, stepping out of our comfort zones opens the door to exciting new friendships.

In this age of social media, it is easy to get caught up in the numbers game of friends and followers. But when it comes to building relationships as we age, quality always trumps quantity. Focus on nurturing deep, meaningful connections with a few close friends and family members who truly understand and support you. These are the relationships that will weather the storms of life and bring endless joy.

You just need to take the time to listen actively, share openly, and express gratitude for the people in your life. Effective communication lays the foundation for strong relationships at any age. Remember, it is not just about talking; it is about truly connecting on a heart-to-heart level. Whether it is a weekly phone call with a loved one or a heartfelt conversation over coffee, make communication a priority.

Life is full of ups and downs, and our relationships are no exception. From disagreements with family members to misunderstandings with friends, challenges are bound to arise. The key is to approach these obstacles with empathy, patience, and a willingness to compromise. Remember, it is okay to agree to disagree sometimes as long as mutual respect remains intact.

Finally, do not forget to prioritize self-care as you navigate the waters of building and maintaining relationships. Just like a garden needs tender love and care to thrive, so do you! Take time for activities that nourish your mind, body, and soul, whether it is practicing yoga, enjoying nature walks, or indulging in your favorite hobbies. When you prioritize your own well-being, you will have even more love and energy to share with those around you.

## The Importance of Social Connections: Finding a Bible-Believing Church and Becoming Involved

Now, let us delve into the significance of social connections within the context of a Bible-believing church community. Finding a spiritual home and becoming actively involved can provide a sense of belonging, purpose, and support that enriches our lives in countless ways. The following sections explore why joining a church and engaging with its members can be a transformative experience as we age.

For many individuals, faith serves as a guiding light throughout their life journey. Joining a church offers a supportive community where we can lean on one another in times of need and rejoice together in times of celebration. Whether facing challenges or experiencing moments of profound gratitude, the fellowship of believers provides a comforting embrace that reminds us we are never alone.

Attending church services, participating in Bible studies, and engaging in worship activities are not only opportunities to connect with others but also avenues for personal spiritual growth. Through the study of scripture, prayer, and fellowship, we deepen our understanding of love and purpose for our lives from God. Surrounding ourselves with fellow believers who share our faith journey encourages us to strive for spiritual excellence and live out our values in meaningful ways.

Church communities are vibrant hubs of diverse individuals united by a common faith. From young families to seasoned elders, people of all ages and backgrounds come together to worship, serve, and grow. Joining a Bible-believing church opens the door to forming deep, lasting relationships with like-minded individuals who share our beliefs and values. These connections go beyond surface-level interactions, fostering friendships rooted in love, trust, and mutual support.

The social connections forged within a church community play a vital role in supporting our mental and emotional well-being. Sharing our joys and burdens with fellow believers creates a sense of solidarity and belonging that lifts our spirits and eases our hearts. Whether through prayer groups, counseling services, or simply lending a listening ear, the caring presence of our church family provides a safe space where we can find solace and strength amidst life's challenges.

One of the most rewarding aspects of church involvement is the opportunity to serve others and make a positive impact in our communities. From volunteering at local shelters to participating in mission trips abroad, churches are actively engaged in outreach efforts that address the physical, emotional, and spiritual needs of those around us. By joining hands with fellow believers in acts of service and compassion, we embody the teachings of Jesus Christ and fulfill our calling to love and serve others selflessly.

From providing a source of strength and comfort to nurturing spiritual growth and fostering deep relationships, church communities play a vital role in supporting our overall well-being and enriching our lives in profound ways. So, if you are searching for a place where you feel you belong and that helps in your growth, consider opening your heart to the transformative power of a loving church family.

## Community Involvement: Finding Purpose in Giving Back Locally

As we age, embracing opportunities to serve others not only strengthens the fabric of our communities but also brings immense fulfillment and joy to our own lives. So, let us dive into the transformative power of community engagement and discover how each of us can make a meaningful difference right where we live.

At the heart of community involvement lies the desire to build stronger, more vibrant neighborhoods where every individual feels valued and supported. Whether it is volunteering at a local soup kitchen, participating in neighborhood clean-up efforts, or mentoring youth in after-school programs, each act of service contributes to the collective well-being of our community. By coming together to address shared challenges and celebrate shared successes, we foster a sense of unity and resilience that uplifts us all.

Every act of kindness, no matter how small, has the power to make a positive impact on the lives of others. From offering a helping hand to a neighbor in need to organizing community events that promote unity and inclusivity, there are countless ways to spread kindness and compassion within our local communities. By stepping outside of ourselves and reaching out to those around us, we create ripple effects of positivity that resonate far beyond our immediate circles.

Engaging in community involvement not only benefits others but also brings profound fulfillment and meaning to our own lives. When we use our time, talents, and resources to serve others, we tap into a deep sense of purpose that transcends the everyday challenges and stresses of life. Whether it is the joy of seeing a smile on the face of someone or the satisfaction of knowing we have made a difference, the rewards of giving back are immeasurable.

Community involvement provides valuable opportunities to connect with individuals from diverse backgrounds and perspectives. By working side by side with fellow volunteers and community members, we forge bonds of friendship and understanding that transcend social barriers and enrich our lives in countless ways. These connections not only strengthen the fabric of our communities but also remind us of the common humanity that unites us all.

As we engage in community involvement, we set a powerful example for future generations to follow. By demonstrating the importance of empathy, compassion, and service, we inspire young people to become active participants in shaping a brighter, more inclusive future for all. Whether it is volunteering as a family or mentoring youth in community programs, we have the opportunity to instill values of kindness and civic responsibility that will echo through the generations to come.

Community involvement offers a profound opportunity to make a positive impact, find purpose, and build stronger, more resilient neighborhoods. Whether through volunteering, advocacy, or simply reaching out to lend a helping hand, each of us has the power to contribute to the greater good right where we live. So, let us embrace the transformative power of community engagement and work together to create a world where kindness, compassion, and solidarity reign supreme.

Here are a few ways you can get involved in your community:

### Environmental Bliss: Unite for a Greener Tomorrow

Join your community in the pursuit of environmental bliss. Embrace the joy of planting trees, not just for shade but as a symbol of growth and renewal. Organize recycling drives that transform waste into opportunities for a cleaner environment. Cultivate community gardens where the soil becomes a canvas for sustainable living, connecting neighbors through the shared love for nature. Together, we can create a tapestry of green, fostering a neighborhood that thrives in harmony with the planet.

## Knowledge Sparks: Illuminate Minds Through Education

Ignite the flames of knowledge within your community. Volunteer your time in tutoring programs, where the spark of understanding lights up young minds. Support adult education classes, providing a pathway to learning for all. Dive into literacy programs, where the magic of words unlocks doors to a brighter future. Your contribution is a beacon, illuminating minds and paving the way for a community that values continuous learning and empowerment.

## Fit and Flourish: Shape a Healthier Lifestyle

Embark on a collective journey toward wellness. Organize fitness classes that transform routine exercise into a celebration of vitality. Host wellness workshops where the secrets of a healthy lifestyle are shared. Contribute to blood drives that sustain life within your community. Build a culture of health together, where each member thrives, radiating positive energy and contributing to the overall well-being of the neighborhood.

### Treasure of Cultures: Celebrate Diversity and Creativity

Become part of a culture that brings your community together. Dive into vibrant cultural events where traditions blend and stories intertwine. Showcase local art exhibitions that paint a picture of diversity and creativity. Participate in performances that resonate with the heartbeat of different backgrounds. Celebrate the richness that each member adds, creating a symphony of cultures that makes your neighborhood truly unique.

### Safety Net: Join Forces for Emergency Response

Become the safety net that holds your community together. Join local emergency response teams, where readiness is the key to swift action. Engage in neighborhood watch programs, where vigilance fosters a secure environment. Your involvement ensures that the threads of safety are woven tightly, creating a fabric that protects and supports every member in times of need.

### Blueprint for Tomorrow: Shape the Destiny of Your Neighborhood

Take an active role in shaping the destiny of your neighborhood. Engage with urban planning and community development committees to chart a course for the future. Collaborate to address specific needs, enhance infrastructure, and create a blueprint that reflects the aspirations of the community. Your involvement is the brushstroke that paints a vision of a thriving and cohesive neighborhood, ensuring a brighter tomorrow for all.

Remember, the key is finding opportunities that align with your interests and skills while addressing the unique needs of your community.

## The Power of Connection: Overcoming Loneliness as We Age

Loneliness is a silent epidemic that can affect anyone, regardless of age, gender, or background. But as we age, its impact can become even more pronounced. Imagine this: you have retired from your job, your children have grown up and moved away, and your circle of friends has dwindled. Suddenly, you find yourself spending more and more time alone, feeling disconnected from the world around you. It is a scenario that many seniors face, and the consequences can be devastating.

But here is the thing: loneliness does not have to define your golden years. In fact, it is never too late to build meaningful connections and reclaim your zest for life.

## The Silent Struggle: Understanding Loneliness

Loneliness goes beyond mere physical isolation; it encompasses a profound sense of emptiness and disconnection that can affect both the mental and physical well-being of an individual. This emotional state often involves feeling misunderstood or uncared for, contributing to a pervasive sense of isolation.

The impact of loneliness on mental health is significant. It can lead to feelings of sadness, anxiety, and even depression. The absence of meaningful connections may leave individuals grappling with a profound sense of purposelessness. The longing for understanding and genuine care can intensify these emotional struggles, creating a cycle that is challenging to break.

On a physical level, loneliness has been linked to various health issues. Chronic loneliness may contribute to increased stress levels, negatively impacting the immune system. Over time, this could make individuals more susceptible to illnesses and other health challenges. Additionally, loneliness might influence lifestyle choices, leading to unhealthy habits that further compromise well-being.

Addressing loneliness involves more than just being around people. It requires cultivating genuine connections and fostering meaningful relationships. Engaging in activities that bring joy and fulfillment can also play a crucial role in combating the pervasive sense of emptiness. Acknowledging and addressing loneliness is an essential step towards enhancing both mental and physical health.

## Breaking the Cycle: Strategies for Connection

The good news is that loneliness is not an inevitable part of aging. There are steps you can take to break free from its grip and cultivate meaningful connections in your life. Here are a few strategies to consider:

### Unlocking Connections: The Power of Taking the First Step

Take the first step in reaching out to people. Building meaningful connections with others is like opening a door to a world of possibilities. One simple and effective way to do this is by taking the first step in reaching out. This could involve joining a local club or community group where shared interests can spark new friendships.

Volunteering is another fantastic avenue to not only give back to the community but also to connect with like-minded individuals. Whether it is contributing to a local charity or participating in environmental initiatives, the shared sense of purpose can create strong bonds.

Sometimes, the key to meaningful connections is right in your neighborhood. Striking up a conversation with a neighbor can be surprisingly rewarding. Whether it is a friendly chat over the fence or a simple "hello" during a walk, small gestures can lead to lasting connections.

Remember, most people are waiting for someone to reach out to them, just like you. By taking that first step, you not only enrich your own life with new connections but also contribute to the vibrant community and friendship around you. So, go ahead, unlock the potential of connection, and discover the joy that comes from reaching out to others.

## Tech-Ties: Nurturing Connections in the Digital Era

In our fast-paced digital age, technology serves as a powerful ally in fostering and maintaining connections. Social media platforms, like Facebook, Instagram, and Twitter, allow you to share snippets of your life and stay updated on the lives of those you care about. It is a virtual window into the worlds of each other, making distance seem less daunting.

Video calls have become a game-changer, bringing face-to-face interactions to the palm of your hand or the screen in front of you. Whether you are catching up with family across the globe or having a virtual coffee date with a friend, the warmth of seeing and hearing loved ones in real-time is unparalleled.

Online forums and communities provide a space for shared interests and passions. Joining groups dedicated to hobbies, professional pursuits, or even specific life experiences opens doors to connecting with individuals who share your enthusiasm. It is a digital avenue to find like-minded souls and build relationships beyond physical boundaries.

Embracing technology in this way not only bridges geographical gaps but also adapts to our busy lives. In the digital realm, staying connected becomes more accessible, making it easier to nurture relationships and weave a digital tapestry of shared moments and meaningful connections.

## Move and Connect: The Dual Benefits of Staying Active

Engaging in physical activity goes beyond keeping your body fit; it is a powerhouse for enhancing mental well-being. Joining a fitness class or adopting a new hobby can be an exciting journey that not only contributes to your physical health but also creates avenues for forging new connections.

Fitness classes, whether at a local gym or through virtual platforms, offer a communal space where individuals come together with a shared goal – staying healthy. The camaraderie developed during workout sessions can extend beyond the gym, providing a foundation for lasting friendships. It is a chance to bond over the shared sweat and triumphs, making the journey toward fitness more enjoyable.

Exploring new hobbies can be a gateway to meeting like-minded individuals. Whether it is a dance class, painting workshop, or hiking group, pursuing interests outside your comfort zone exposes you to a diverse range of people. Shared passions form a solid foundation for connections, turning acquaintances into friends who understand and appreciate the joy your chosen activity brings.

Remember, staying active is not just about physical exertion; it is an investment in your holistic well-being. As you embark on the path of physical activity, you are not only taking care of your body but also opening doors to a world of potential friendships and connections that enrich your life in more ways than one.

## Gratitude: A Simple Practice for a Richer Life

Cultivating an attitude of gratitude can be a transformative journey that redirects your focus from what you lack to the abundance that surrounds you. Taking a few moments each day to reflect on the things you are grateful for has the power to elevate your mood and enhance your overall well-being.

Consider starting a gratitude journal. It does not have to be elaborate; a simple notebook will do. Each day, jot down a few things you are thankful for. It could be the warmth of sunlight streaming through your window, a delicious meal, or a kind gesture from a colleague. This practice helps you actively acknowledge and appreciate the positive aspects of your life.

Gratitude not only influences your mindset but also deepens your connections with others. Expressing appreciation to friends, family, or colleagues for their support or kindness strengthens your relationships. People often cherish being recognized for their contributions, and your gratitude can create a positive ripple effect in your social circles.

As you make gratitude a daily habit, you will likely find that your perspective shifts, making room for more joy and contentment. Embracing the simple act of appreciating the small moments and blessings in your life can be a powerful tool in fostering a positive outlook and nurturing meaningful connections with those around you.

## Reaching Out for Support: Embracing Professional Guidance

If you find yourself grappling with persistent feelings of loneliness, reaching out to a mental health professional can be a crucial step toward healing. Therapists and counselors are skilled professionals equipped to offer valuable support and guidance as you navigate through the complexities of loneliness.

Opening up to a professional about your emotions provides a safe space to explore the root causes of your loneliness. They can help you identify patterns of thought and behavior that may contribute to your feelings of isolation, offering insights and coping strategies tailored to your unique situation.

The therapeutic journey is a collaborative process. Your therapist or counselor becomes a partner in your quest for emotional well-being. They offer a non-judgmental ear, helping you unpack and understand your emotions. Through this process, you can gain a deeper insight into yourself, fostering personal growth and resilience.

Remember, seeking professional help is a sign of strength, not weakness. Loneliness is a common human experience, and professionals are trained to provide the tools and support needed to overcome it. Taking this step not only prioritizes your mental health but also empowers you to build a stronger foundation for meaningful connections and a more fulfilling life.

Ultimately, overcoming loneliness is about recognizing the power of connection in our lives. By reaching out to others, embracing new experiences, and staying engaged in the world around us, we can build a support network that sustains us through the ups and downs of life.

So, as you navigate the journey of aging, remember this: you are never truly alone. There are people out there who care about you and want to see you thrive. By taking proactive steps to nurture your connections, you can create a life filled with meaning, purpose, and joy—no matter what your age may be.

DONALD WEST

*"Forbearing one another, and forgiving one another, if any man have a quarrel against any: even as Christ forgave you, so also do ye."*

*- Colossians 3:13 KJV*

# Chapter 5
# Preventive Health-Care

As we grow older, taking care of our health becomes even more important. One key aspect of staying healthy is making sure to have regular check-ups with your doctor. These routine medical examinations are important to keep a health check over your body and help catch potential issues early on, keeping you on the path to a happy and healthy life.

Seniors may not always feel sick, but routine check-ups can spot hidden problems. Just like a superhero detecting trouble before it strikes, doctors can find issues early on. This can include issues like high blood pressure, diabetes, or even signs of major health problems like cancer. Early detection means easier solutions and a better chance of staying healthy.

Sometimes, seniors have health needs that are different from those of younger people. Routine check-ups help doctors keep track of changes in health over time. By understanding these trends, they can adjust care plans and provide personalized advice to keep seniors feeling their best.

Health is not just about the body; it is also about the mind. Routine check-ups provide an opportunity for seniors to discuss any emotional or mental health concerns. At times, seniors may feel lonely, stressed, or anxious, and discussing these emotions during check-ups is crucial. Healthcare professionals are there to help, offering support and guidance. Addressing emotional or mental health concerns early on can make a significant difference in the overall well-being of a senior.

Seniors often face unique challenges, such as adjusting to retirement, loss of loved ones, or health-related issues. These challenges can take a toll on their mental health. Regular check-ups create a safe space for seniors to express their concerns and receive appropriate care or referrals to specialists if needed.

Mental well-being automatically contributes to a more enjoyable life. When emotional health is prioritized, seniors may find it easier to engage in activities they love, connect with others, and maintain a positive outlook on life. With this, they foster a holistic approach to health that encompasses both physical and mental aspects. So, addressing these issues early on can lead to better overall well-being and a more enjoyable life.

Most importantly, seeing the same doctor regularly helps build a strong, trusting relationship. Seniors can feel more comfortable discussing their health concerns, and doctors can provide personalized care based on a deep understanding of the health history of the individual.

So, routine medical examinations are like a superhero team for the health of seniors – detecting problems early, managing chronic conditions, ensuring proper medication, supporting emotional well-being, and building strong doctor-patient relationships. By prioritizing these check-ups, seniors can enjoy a healthier, happier life.

## Why Regular Check-Ups Matter

Here are a few ways as to why regular checkups are essential for your body:

### 1. Early Detection of Health Issues:

As discussed above, regular check-ups allow your doctor to detect any health problems at an early stage. This is crucial because many health conditions can be more effectively treated when identified at the initial stages.

### 2. Preventing Serious Complications:

By identifying and addressing health concerns early on, you can prevent more serious complications from developing. Regular check-ups act as a preventive measure, helping you maintain a good quality of life.

### 3. Managing Chronic Conditions:

For seniors with chronic conditions like diabetes or hypertension, regular check-ups are essential for monitoring and managing these conditions. This helps in adjusting medications and lifestyle factors to keep these conditions under control.

### 4. Vaccinations and Immunizations:

Seniors may need certain vaccinations or immunizations to protect against diseases. Regular check-ups provide an opportunity for your doctor to discuss and administer these vaccines, ensuring you stay protected.

### 5. Medication Review:

As we age, the medications we take may need adjustments. Regular check-ups allow your doctor to review your medications, ensuring they are still appropriate and not causing any adverse effects.

### 6. Mental Health Check:

Mental health is just as important as physical health. Regular check-ups provide an opportunity for your doctor to discuss any mental health concerns, offering support or referrals to specialists if needed.

## Build the Mighty Castle of Your Body: Tips for Staying Healthy

Let us explore the key battlements that you need to fortify to stay healthy.

### Fuel up with Powerful Potions:

Imagine your plate as a magic spell book full of tasty tricks! Add colorful fruits and veggies like the colorful spells in your book—they come in different shapes and sizes, each with its unique power, like red peppers give you a vitamin C boost. Lean proteins are your muscle-building allies, giving you the strength to tackle any quest. Whole grains are energy wizards, keeping you charged up throughout the day. Healthy fats are regarded as the best friends for the brain, helping you think sharp and smart.

Throw in lean proteins for strong muscles, and do not forget the whole grains and healthy fats; they are the secret ingredients for energy and brainpower.

This mix is a potion that will guide you against illness and make you feel unstoppable.

## Exercise: Your Daily Dose of Dragon-Slaying:

Think of staying active as having your own loyal dragon companion—it is a fun adventure! No need for swords; just find activities you enjoy. A brisk walk in the park or a splash in the water (like a friendly swim) are perfect quests. Even gentle stretches are the magic spells that keep your body feeling young and strong.

Your heart then becomes a powerful fortress, ready for any battle life throws at you. So, gear up, grab your invisible sword (or not), and let the daily dragon-slaying begin!

## Sleep: The Nightly Guardian of Your Castle

Just as a sturdy moat safeguards a castle, ensuring you get 7-8 hours of quality sleep each night acts as a protective shield for your body. Sleep serves as a magical recharge, fortifying your bodily defenses and leaving you feeling refreshed and ready to take on the challenges of the day. During sleep, your body repairs itself, and your mind consolidates memories, making it a crucial element in maintaining overall well-being.

Creating a bedtime routine can enhance the quality of your sleep. Dim the lights, avoid screen time before bed, and relax with a calming activity. These habits contribute to a restful night time sleep, allowing your body to reap the full benefits of its nightly restoration process.

### Hygiene: The Invisible Moat Against Invaders

Regular handwashing, particularly before meals and after being in public places, is similar to raising a drawbridge to block those pesky germs from entering your body. It is a simple yet powerful defense strategy to stay healthy and prevent the spread of illnesses.

Maintaining personal hygiene through regular showers and clean clothes creates an additional layer of protection. Just as a well-kept moat deters invaders, a clean and hygienic lifestyle helps keep germs at bay, ensuring you can go about your day feeling confident and resilient.

### Sun Protection: Your Shield Against Ultraviolet Dragons:

The sun might seem friendly, but its ultraviolet rays can be like fire-breathing dragons for your skin. To safeguard the well-being of your skin, consider constructing a robust sun shield. Start by diligently applying a broad-spectrum sunscreen, creating a protective barrier against harmful UV rays. Complement this with the strategic use of clothing that shields your skin from direct sun exposure.

Timing is crucial, so avoid venturing out during the midday sun, when the fiery breath of the dragon is most intense. By fortifying your defenses, you can ensure your skin remains not only healthy but resilient against the relentless assault of ultraviolet dragons.

## Mental & Emotional Well-being: Your Inner Strength:

Beyond the realm of physical health, nurturing your mental and emotional well-being is equally important. Discovering activities that bring you joy and fulfillment contributes to the construction of a robust inner wall. Whether it is pursuing hobbies, engaging in mindfulness practices, or embracing creative endeavors, these acts of self-care bolster the foundations of your mental resilience.

Strengthening your inner wall extends to maintaining connections with loved ones and fostering a support network that acts as an impervious shield against life challenges. When the fortress faces adversity, do not hesitate to seek support, for it is in unity that the inner strength becomes unbreakable. In the fortress of your mind and spirit, you hold the power to withstand the storms of life, emerging with an enduring sense of well-being.

Remember, building your health fortress is a continuous journey. By incorporating these simple yet powerful tips into your daily routine, you can empower your body to stay strong and healthy, ensuring a fulfilling and vibrant life as you age. So, grab your metaphorical sword and shield, and let us conquer the path to wellness together!

## Maintaining Chronic Conditions: Living Well with Age-Related Health Issues

Age often brings with it a collection of chronic conditions such as arthritis, diabetes, heart disease, and more. Rather than viewing these as roadblocks, seniors can consider them as unique chapters in their life stories, each requiring a unique and tailored approach for effective management.

Managing chronic conditions requires a blend of patience, understanding, and a commitment to holistic well-being. Acceptance is the first step towards a fulfilling life. Embrace the changes that come with time, acknowledging that each day is a new chapter. Understand that your body is a resilient companion, and with proper care, it can flourish even in the face of challenges.

You need to surround yourself with a network of care and understanding. Share your experiences with loved ones, creating an open conversation about your health. A support system not only eases the burden but also fosters an environment where love and empathy thrive.

Caring for yourself goes beyond medical treatments. Nourish your body with wholesome foods, engage in gentle exercises, and prioritize adequate rest. Seek activities that bring joy and purpose, whether it is pursuing hobbies, spending time with loved ones, or simply enjoying the beauty of nature.

It is important to develop a strong partnership with your healthcare team. Knowledge is power. Take the time to comprehend your health condition. Consult with your healthcare provider, ask questions, and seek clarification. Understanding the ins and outs of your ailment empowers you to make informed decisions about your well-being.

Chronic conditions can even take a toll on mental health. Cultivate mindfulness through practices like meditation or deep breathing. Stay socially connected, and if needed, seek the support of mental health professionals. Emotional well-being is an integral part of aging gracefully with chronic conditions.

A positive mindset acts as a beacon of light during the journey of managing chronic conditions. Seniors can choose to focus on what they can control, celebrate small victories, and cultivate gratitude. This mindset shift is akin to turning challenges into opportunities for growth and resilience.

Just as a seasoned sailor acknowledges the unpredictability of the sea, seniors can cheerfully accept certain limitations that come with age-related health issues. But you need not give up; instead, find new ways to enjoy life. This might involve adapting activities, seeking support when needed, and exploring new interests that align with current capabilities.

Navigating your life journey is not a solo expedition. You need to cultivate a supportive network of friends, family, and community. This network is like a safety net, providing encouragement, understanding, and assistance when facing the inevitable challenges that come with chronic conditions.

Living well with age-related health issues involves finding purpose and joy in daily life. Seniors can explore activities that bring fulfillment, whether it is pursuing hobbies, volunteering, or spending quality time with loved ones. This purposeful living is the wind in their sails, propelling them forward with enthusiasm.

Remember, managing chronic conditions is an art of living well despite health challenges. You can navigate this journey with grace, collaborating with healthcare providers, adhering to medications, embracing lifestyle modifications, maintaining a positive mindset, cheerfully accepting limitations, building a supportive network, and engaging in purposeful living. By steering your ship with wisdom and resilience, you can find joy and fulfillment in each chapter of your unique life story.

*"Beloved, I wish above all things that thou mayest prosper and be in health, even as thy soul prospereth."*

*- 3 John 2 KJV*

# Chapter 6

# Hobbies and Passions

Life is a beautiful journey with seasons of change and growth. Just like the changing landscapes outside, our interests and passions can evolve throughout our lives. As we enter our senior years, a new chapter unfolds, presenting a wonderful opportunity to explore, discover, and cultivate new interests that spark joy and fulfillment.

Retirement can be a wonderful time! It is a chance to say goodbye to the daily work routine and hello to more freedom and fun. You can finally focus on all the things you enjoy, whether it is spending time with loved ones, traveling to new places, or picking up a long-forgotten hobby.

However, with all that free time, it is natural to feel a little lost sometimes. You might wonder what to do with yourself after years of following a set schedule. This feeling of "What now?" is completely normal. It is just your mind adjusting to this big change.

The good news is that this is your chance to explore! You can try new things, reconnect with old passions, or simply relax and enjoy the slower pace of life. There are endless possibilities – the key is to find what brings you a sense of purpose and fulfillment.

The world is brimming with exciting possibilities. From mastering a new language to delving into the world of art, there is something out there for everyone. In these years of life, cultivating interests becomes a delightful journey that brings joy, fulfillment, and a sense of purpose. Seniors, like anyone else, deserve the richness of diverse experiences, and pursuing hobbies is a wonderful way to achieve that.

Just like the changing seasons, it is perfectly alright to have hobbies that are enjoyed for a specific time. Perhaps you have always wanted to learn a musical instrument, and now is the time to do so. Embracing seasonal hobbies allows for variety, preventing monotony and adding spice to life. The key is to find what sparks that inner joy and excitement.

Some hobbies become lifelong companions, offering continuous fulfillment. Reading, for instance, is a timeless hobby that transports you to different worlds through the pages of a book. Engaging in activities like birdwatching, yoga, or joining a community club can provide lasting joy and a sense of belonging.

Having a mix of hobbies adds flavor to each day. Consider rotating between creative ideas, physical activities, and intellectual endeavors. This variety not only keeps life interesting but also contributes to maintaining a healthy and balanced lifestyle.

Cultivating interests is not just a solo endeavor; it is an opportunity to connect with others. Joining clubs or groups with shared interests fosters social connections, providing a support system and a platform for exchanging ideas and experiences.

Here are some tips to help you ignite the spark of interest:

**Think back:** Reflect on activities you enjoyed in the past, perhaps from your younger years or even your career. Did you find joy in painting, playing an instrument, or gardening? Rekindle those passions and see if they still resonate with you.

**Explore your surroundings:** Take a stroll through your local museum, library, or community center. Often, these places offer a variety of activities and classes specifically designed for seniors. You might discover a hidden talent or rediscover a long-forgotten passion.

**Chat with friends and family:** Talk to loved ones about their hobbies and interests. You might be surprised by what you learn and discover a shared passion you can explore together.

**Do not be afraid to try new things**: Stepping outside your comfort zone can lead to wonderful discoveries. Sign up for a beginner-level class in something that piques your curiosity, whether it is photography, dancing, or creative writing. You might just surprise yourself with hidden talents and newfound joy.

As with any journey, there may be obstacles along the way. Physical limitations or health concerns might pose challenges, but adapting hobbies to suit your abilities ensures that the joy of pursuing interests remains undiminished. Seek assistance when needed, and explore modified versions of your favorite activities.

So, embark on this adventure, savor the moments, and let the richness of diverse interests enhance the experience of your golden years.

## Embracing Lifelong Learning: Keeping Your Mind Sharp and Engaged

Imagine yourself, years from now, still vibrant and curious, tackling new challenges and experiences. This is not just wishful thinking; it is the reality that awaits those who embrace lifelong learning. As we age, our bodies may change, but our minds hold the incredible potential to keep growing and evolving. Just like our bodies benefit from staying active, so do our brains thrive when we engage in stimulating activities that keep them sharp and engaged.

While many associate learning with classrooms and textbooks, the truth is lifelong learning is a crucial aspect of a fulfilling life at any age. It is about keeping your mind active, expanding your knowledge, and enriching your experiences throughout your golden years. Just like the pages of a book turn, life offers opportunities to delve into new experiences, gaining knowledge and wisdom along the way. Embracing the spirit of lifelong learning adds vibrancy to each day.

Think about it this way: our brains are like muscles. The more you use them, the stronger and more resilient they become. Conversely, if left unused, they can weaken over time. Lifelong learning is similar to a regular workout for your brain, building cognitive strength and keeping it nimble and adaptable.

This is not just about staving off age-related decline. Studies have shown that engaging in lifelong learning offers a plethora of benefits for seniors, including:

## Boost Your Brainpower: Unlock the Benefits of Learning!

Ever wonder why learning a new skill or picking up a new hobby feels so good? It is not just about the fun or the accomplishment. It is actually giving your brain a workout, and just like any other muscle, the more you challenge it, the stronger it gets!

When you learn something new, your brain forms new connections between brain cells. Learning often involves figuring things out and overcoming challenges. This constant mental exercise strengthens your problem-solving skills, making you better equipped to tackle any obstacle that comes your way.

## Unlocking Happiness: How Learning New Things Can Uplift Your Mood

Imagine the feeling of finally mastering a challenging skill, like cooking that perfect dish or speaking a few phrases in a new language. This sense of accomplishment is like a gold medal for your brain, boosting your self-esteem and making you feel more confident in taking on new challenges. It is like saying, "I did this, so I can definitely do that too!"

Learning new things can boost self-esteem and confidence, providing a sense of accomplishment and purpose. It can also combat feelings of boredom and isolation, leading to a more positive outlook on life. So, next time you are feeling down or uninspired, remember that learning is more than just acquiring knowledge; it is a key to unlocking happiness and a more fulfilling life!

## Learning Together, Growing Together: How Learning Strengthens Your Social Circle

Learning does not have to be a solo adventure! In fact, joining forces with others to explore new knowledge can be a fantastic way to strengthen your social connections. Stepping outside your comfort zone and learning something new alongside others opens doors to meeting new people who share similar interests.

Whether you are taking a pottery class or joining a book club, these shared experiences create a natural foundation for conversation and connection. You never know who you might click with, and a shared passion for learning can blossom into lasting friendships.

To benefit from learning, one delightful way to keep the mind agile is by exploring new genres of literature. If you have always been a fan of mysteries, why not venture into the world of historical fiction? If romance novels are your usual go-to, consider trying science fiction for a change. Diversifying your reading habits introduces fresh perspectives and sparks intellectual curiosity.

Engaging in creative activities, such as writing short stories or poetry, is a wonderful form of lifelong learning. It allows you to express thoughts and emotions while challenging the mind to think creatively. Do not worry about perfection; the joy lies in the process of self-expression and exploration.

The digital era has brought learning to your fingertips. Online courses and workshops cover a myriad of subjects, from history and science to art and technology. Platforms like Coursera, Khan Academy, or even local community centers offer opportunities to learn at your own pace. Choose topics that ignite your curiosity and open doors to new knowledge.

Technology is not just for the younger generation; it is a valuable tool for seniors, too. Dive into the world of podcasts, audiobooks, and educational apps. These resources provide a convenient way to learn on the go, whether you are taking a stroll, relaxing at home, or commuting. The possibilities are endless.

Attend concerts, visit museums, or explore local art galleries. Immersing yourself in the arts stimulates the mind and introduces you to different cultures and perspectives. Learn about different art forms, from classical music to contemporary art, and let the creative expressions of others inspire you.

Engaging in conversations with others is a powerful way to learn and share ideas. Joining book clubs or discussion groups, either in person or online, creates a space for intellectual exchange. It exposes you to diverse viewpoints and enriches your understanding of various topics.

Curiosity is the fuel for lifelong learning. Ask questions, seek answers, and never stop wondering. Whether it is exploring the wonders of nature, learning about scientific advancements, or understanding historical events, the quest for knowledge keeps the mind vibrant and youthful.

## Keeping Your Mind Active: A World of Possibilities:

The bright side of it is that lifelong learning can take many forms, and there is no single "right" way to do it. Here are some ways to keep your mind engaged:

**Embrace the world of reading**: As discussed above, dive into a genre you have not explored before – delve into historical biographies, lose yourself in captivating science fiction, or explore the depths of philosophical thought. Reading exposes you to new ideas, perspectives, and information, stimulating your mind and imagination.

**Become a lifelong learner:** Enroll in a local community college course, take an online learning program, or join a lecture series. The options are endless, from mastering a new language to learning about local history or exploring the wonders of astronomy.

**Engage in creative pursuits**: Unleash your creativity through activities like painting, writing, photography, or even learning to play a musical instrument. Engaging in creative activities stimulates different parts of the brain, enhancing cognitive function and providing a sense of joy and self-expression.

**Challenge yourself with puzzles and games:** Crossword puzzles, Sudoku, brain teasers, and jigsaw puzzles are excellent ways to keep your mind sharp and improve problem-solving skills. They are also a fun way to pass the time and can even be enjoyed with friends and family.

**Engage in stimulating conversations:** Surround yourself with people who inspire you and challenge your thinking. Engage in meaningful conversations about current events, philosophy, or even everyday life. Learning from others and expanding your understanding of the world keeps your mind active and engaged.

Lifelong learning is a journey that breathes life into each passing day. By exploring new genres, embracing technology, and engaging in creative pursuits, you foster a sense of curiosity and intellectual vitality. So, embark on this lifelong learning adventure, and let the joy of discovering new experiences keep your mind forever young.

## Creative Outlets: Expressing Yourself Through Art, Music, or Writing

As we age, life can sometimes take unexpected turns. Retirement, changes in health, and even the loss of loved ones can leave us feeling a bit lost, searching for new ways to fill our days with meaning and purpose. But amidst these changes lies a beautiful opportunity: the chance to rediscover the joy and power of creativity.

For many seniors, the golden years present a unique opportunity to tap into their creativity and express themselves through various artistic mediums

– be it the vibrant colors of a canvas, the soothing melodies of music, or the captivating power of words.

You might be wondering, "Why is creativity so important, especially at this stage of life?" Well, the answer is simple: Creativity is a wonderful gift that allows us to express our thoughts, emotions, and unique perspectives. Engaging in creative outlets like art, music, or writing provides a channel for self-expression and a means to communicate without words.

You do not need to be a professional artist to enjoy the benefits of creating art. Whether it is painting, drawing, or even doodling, art allows you to visually convey your feelings. Experiment with different mediums and styles, embracing the freedom to express yourself without judgment.

The essence of creative expression is not perfection but the authenticity of your voice. Embrace imperfections and view each creation as a unique piece of your journey. Let go of the pressure to be flawless, and enjoy the process of self-discovery through your creative outlets.

Creative outlets are pathways to self-discovery and joy. Whether you are painting a canvas, strumming a guitar, or penning your thoughts, each creative endeavor is a celebration of your unique spirit.

## Exploring the Artistic World:

The world of art is vast and welcoming, offering something for everyone. Here are a few ideas to get your creative juices flowing:

- **Painting and drawing**: Whether you are a seasoned artist or a complete beginner, there are endless possibilities. Experiment with watercolors, acrylics, pastels, or even charcoal. You can join a class, find inspiration online, or simply grab a sketchbook and start doodling.

- **Sculpting**: Molding clay into forms, big or small, can be a therapeutic and rewarding experience. It allows you to express yourself in a three-dimensional way and explore your sense of touch and texture.

- **Crafting**: From knitting and crocheting to jewelry making and woodworking, the world of crafts offers something for everyone. It is a great way to create unique and beautiful objects while also engaging your fine motor skills.

## Finding Your Voice Through Music:

Music is a universal language that can evoke a wide range of emotions. Whether you have always dreamed of playing an instrument or simply enjoy singing along to your favorite tunes, here are some ways to embrace music in your life:

- **Learn a new instrument:** It is never too late to pick up a guitar, piano, or even an ukulele! Many community centers and music schools offer classes specifically designed for older adults.

- **Join a choir or singing group:** Singing in a group is a wonderful way to connect with others, learn new songs, and experience the joy of creating beautiful music together.

- **Attend concerts and musical events:** Immerse yourself in the world of music by attending live performances. It is a great way to stay connected to your favorite artists and discover new ones.

## The Power of the Written Word:

Writing is a powerful tool for self-expression, reflection, and storytelling. Whether you choose to write poems, short stories, or even a memoir, here are some ways to get started:

- **Join a writing group:** Sharing your work with others in a supportive environment can be incredibly motivating and helpful. Many libraries and community centers offer writing workshops and groups specifically for seniors.

- **Start a personal journal:** Journaling is a wonderful way to document your thoughts, feelings, and experiences. It can be a space for self-reflection, exploration, and creative expression.

- **Write for online communities:** There are many online platforms where you can share your writing with others who have common interests with you. This can be a great way to connect with a wider audience and receive feedback on your work.

**Remember:**

1. Do not worry about being perfect: Just have fun and enjoy the process of learning and creating.
2. You do not need experience: There are classes and resources available for beginners of all ages.
3. Look for inspiration: Find things you like in the world around you and use them as ideas for your own creations.
4. Share your work: Show your creations to friends and family, or even enter them in local contests.

By trying new things and expressing yourself in different ways, you can add joy and meaning to your life. So, express yourself freely, explore different forms of creativity, and let your imagination flow as you embark on this artistic journey of self-expression.

*"Whatsoever thy hand findeth to do, do it with thy might; for there is no work, nor device, nor knowledge, nor wisdom, in the grave, whither thou goest."*

*- Ecclesiastes 9:10 KJV*

# Chapter 7
# Financial Wellness

Retirement is a well-deserved break after years of hard work. It is a time to pursue hobbies, travel, and spend time with loved ones. But before you pack your bags and hit the beach, it is crucial to think about your finances. In this chapter, we will explore the key considerations for seniors when navigating the financial aspects of retirement.

Planning for retirement can feel overwhelming, especially when it comes to finances. First, take a deep breath and remember that you do not have to do this alone. There are many resources available to help you with retirement planning, like financial advisors, senior centers, and even government agencies. Do not hesitate to reach out for help and guidance – that is what they are there for!

Next, break down the big picture into smaller, more manageable pieces. Instead of trying to figure out everything at once, focus on one step at a time. There are different aspects to consider, like your income sources, your expected expenses, and how much you have saved up so far. Take some time to gather your information and get a clear understanding of your current financial situation.

Even small steps can make a big difference. Once you have a better handle on your finances, you can start making informed decisions about your retirement. Do not be discouraged if it takes some time and effort – creating a secure and comfortable retirement is definitely worth the investment.

Before diving into numbers, take a moment to envision your ideal retirement. What does your lifestyle look like? Do you see yourself staying in your current home, downsizing, or living in a retirement community? Are there travel destinations you have always wanted to visit? Having a clear picture of your desired lifestyle will help you determine your financial needs.

Take a close look at your income and expenses. How much are you bringing in from pensions, Social Security, or other sources? What are your regular monthly expenses, including housing, utilities, groceries, and healthcare? Knowing where your money stands will give you a realistic picture of your financial starting point.

Once you have a grasp of your income and expenses, create a budget specifically for your retirement. This will help you track your spending and ensure you stay within your means. Be sure to factor in potential future costs like healthcare, travel, and long-term care. Remember, inflation is a real factor, so try to build in some flexibility in your budget to account for rising costs over time.

If you have not already, it is never too late to start saving for retirement. Consider contributing to employer-sponsored retirement plans, like 401(k)s or individual retirement accounts (IRAs). These accounts offer tax advantages that can significantly boost your savings over time. Take advantage of any employer matching contributions to free up extra money for retirement savings.

Do not put all your eggs in one basket! Diversifying your investment portfolio across different asset classes like stocks, bonds, and real estate can help you manage risk and potentially increase your returns. As you approach retirement, you may want to gradually shift your portfolio towards more conservative investments to protect your principal.

## Supercharge Your Retirement Savings

Once you have a handle on your income and expenses, create a realistic budget. This will help you track your spending and ensure your income covers your needs throughout your retirement. Remember, unexpected expenses can pop up, so consider building a buffer into your budget with an emergency fund that covers 3-6 months of living expenses.

Here are some strategies to stretch your retirement dollars:

### Boost Your Nest Egg with Every Paycheck:

Many employers offer matching contributions to your retirement savings plan, essentially adding free money to your account. Do not miss out on this valuable benefit! Increase your contributions to reach the employer match threshold and watch your retirement savings soar.

The power of compound interest is on your side when you start saving early. Even small contributions made regularly can accumulate significantly over time. Make saving for retirement a priority from the beginning of your career.

### Do not Play Catch-Up: Contribute More If You are over 50

If you are over 50, you are eligible to make additional contributions to your retirement accounts beyond the standard limits. This is a fantastic opportunity to accelerate your savings and make up for any lost ground if you start saving later in life.

Take advantage of catch-up contributions to significantly boost your retirement nest egg. Remember, the sooner you start saving, the more time your money has to grow.

## Weather the Storm: Review and Adjust Your Investment Portfolio

As you near retirement, your risk tolerance may shift. Consider gradually reducing your exposure to volatile assets like stocks and increasing your investments in more stable options like bonds. This can help protect your savings from market fluctuations and provide peace of mind as you approach retirement.

While this general advice offers a starting point, consulting with a qualified financial advisor is crucial. They can assess your individual circumstances, risk tolerance, and retirement goals to create a personalized investment strategy tailored to your unique needs.

In addition to retirement savings and Social Security, you may want to consider other options to supplement your income in retirement. This could include part-time work, renting out a room in your home, or starting a small business.

Planning for retirement is an ongoing process. Regularly review your budget, investments, and overall financial situation to ensure you are on track to achieve your retirement goals. By taking proactive steps and making informed decisions, you can navigate the financial considerations of retirement and pave the way for a happy and fulfilling golden age.

## Understanding and Preparing for Medical Expenses in Retirement

Health is a treasure, and as we step into retirement, it is essential to understand and prepare for medical expenses. With age comes an increased need for medical services, making it crucial to understand and prepare for these expenses to avoid financial strain in retirement. Healthcare is an essential part of life, and its costs can be a significant concern, especially for seniors planning their retirement.

Healthcare costs are generally higher for seniors compared to younger adults due to several factors. These include the increased likelihood of chronic health conditions, the need for preventive care and regular checkups, and the potential for needing more complex medical services like surgeries or hospitalizations. Additionally, the cost of prescription medications and long-term care can add up significantly.

### Understanding Your Insurance Options:

**Medicare:** The government-funded program provides health insurance for most Americans aged

65 and over, as well as younger individuals with certain disabilities. Medicare has two main parts:

Part A: Covers hospital stays, skilled nursing facility care, hospice care, and home healthcare in some cases.

Part B: Covers doctor visits, outpatient services, some preventive care, and durable medical equipment.

Medicare Supplement (Medigap) Plans: These private insurance plans help cover out-of-pocket costs associated with Original Medicare, such as deductibles, copayments, and coinsurance.

Medicare Part D: This optional program provides coverage for prescription drugs.

It is important to remember that Medicare does not cover everything. You may still have out-of-pocket expenses, such as deductibles, copayments, and coinsurance. Additionally, Medicare does not cover dental care, vision care, or long-term care services.[1]

---

[1] https://www.medicare.gov/

Here are the strategies for Managing Costs:

## Empower Yourself with Knowledge:

**Become a Medicare Master:** Do not let the alphabet soup of Medicare confuse you. Take the time to understand the different parts (A, B, C, and D) and their coverage. This knowledge empowers you to make informed decisions about your healthcare needs and financial future.

**Decode Your Insurance Options**: Explore the various Medicare Supplement and Part D plans available in your area. Each plan offers unique benefits and costs, so deciphering this information is crucial to finding the perfect fit for your budget and health requirements.

## Become a Comparison Champion:

**Shop Around Like a Pro:** Do not fall into the trap of choosing the first plan you encounter. Utilize online resources or seek guidance from a licensed insurance agent to compare various plans. This proactive approach ensures you select the most cost-effective and beneficial option for your specific situation.

**Negotiate Like a Boss:** Do not shy away from negotiating! Healthcare costs can be substantial, so do not hesitate to discuss fees with medical providers or negotiate prescription drug prices. A little conversation can go a long way in saving you money.

## Unlock the Secrets to Savings:

**Generic Gems:** Embrace the power of generic medications. They offer the same effectiveness as brand-name drugs but at a significantly lower cost. Talk to your doctor about the possibility of switching to generic medications when appropriate.

**Discount Drug Detectives:** Explore discount programs and prescription savings cards offered by various providers or organizations. These programs can offer significant savings on your medication costs, so take advantage of them!

## Plan for the Long Haul:

**Safeguard Your Future:** Long-term care expenses can quickly deplete your savings. Consider investing in long-term care insurance to protect yourself from these potentially overwhelming costs.

**Explore Alternative Avenues:** Research alternative options to traditional long-term care facilities. In-home care services or modifications to your living space can offer a more affordable and comfortable solution for some individuals.

By following these comprehensive strategies, you can effectively manage your medical expenses in retirement, ensuring financial security and peace of mind as you navigate this new chapter in your life.

Do not hesitate to seek help from professionals like financial advisors, healthcare advocates, or social workers. They can provide valuable guidance on navigating the complexities of healthcare costs and managing your resources effectively.

By understanding your options, planning for potential costs, and taking proactive steps to manage your finances, you can take control of your healthcare costs in retirement and focus on enjoying your golden years with peace of mind.

## Finding Your Golden Nest: Selecting a Senior Residence That Combines Comfort and Support

As we age, our needs and preferences evolve. While the spacious family home served you well for years, it might not be the ideal environment in your later years. You may consider downsizing to a more manageable space, offering easier access to assistance and fostering a sense of community.

The first and most crucial step is self-reflection. What are your present and anticipated physical abilities? Do you foresee needing any assistance with daily tasks like bathing, dressing, or preparing meals? Consider your desired level of social interaction; do you thrive in a vibrant environment with planned activities, or would you prefer a quieter setting? Thinking about these aspects will help you narrow down your search and find a residence that aligns with your individual needs and preferences.

When considering our later residence, let us focus on a few key aspects that can make this transition smoother and more enjoyable. First and foremost, think about location. Opt for a place that is close to essential services, like hospitals, pharmacies, and grocery stores. This way, help is readily available, and you would not feel cut off from the resources you need.

A senior-friendly community can make a significant difference. Look for residences that prioritize accessibility, with ramps, elevators, and other features that make mobility easier. Such communities often foster a sense of belonging, providing opportunities to socialize and engage with others.

Safety is another paramount concern. Ensure that the chosen residence has security measures in place, such as well-lit areas and 24/7 monitoring. Feeling secure in our living environment is vital for peace of mind and overall well-being.

Consider the level of assistance available. Some senior residences offer a range of support services, from basic aid with daily activities to more intensive medical care. Assess your current and potential future needs to select a residence that can accommodate those needs as they evolve.

Amenities and recreational activities should not be overlooked. Choose a residence that provides opportunities for social interaction, exercise, and leisure. This ensures a vibrant and engaging lifestyle, preventing feelings of isolation and promoting a sense of community.

Affordability is a practical aspect that cannot be ignored. Carefully assess your budget and explore options that align with your financial situation. Do not hesitate to inquire about any available financial assistance programs or subsidies that could make your chosen residence more affordable.

### Making the Decision:

**Visit and research**: Do not be afraid to visit different communities and ask questions. Talk to residents and staff, get a feel for the atmosphere, and see if it is a place you can picture yourself living in. Read online reviews and compare available options based on your needs and budget.

**Talk to family and friends:** Involve your loved ones in the decision-making process. Seek their advice and support as you explore different options.

**Do not rush:** Finding the right senior living option is a big decision. Take your time, weigh your options carefully, and choose a place that feels comfortable and secure for you and your future needs.

## Leaving a Legacy: Planning for the Secured Future of Your Loved Ones

As we age, our thoughts naturally turn towards the future and the well-being of those we care about most. Legacy planning is the process of making thoughtful decisions about how you want your assets, values, and experiences to be passed on to future generations. It goes beyond simply dividing your belongings - it is about expressing your love, ensuring financial security for your loved ones, and leaving a positive and lasting impact.

Legacy is more than just material possessions. It encompasses your values, experiences, and the impact you have made on the world. Before delving into legal and financial aspects, consider what you want your legacy to be. Do you want to be remembered for your kindness, generosity, or humor? Do you value family traditions and want to ensure they continue? Identifying your core values will guide your decisions throughout the legacy planning process.

## Key Elements of Legacy Planning:

**Estate Planning:** This involves creating legal documents like wills, trusts, and powers of attorney. These documents outline your wishes regarding the distribution of your assets, appoint individuals responsible for managing your affairs, and define how you want your healthcare decisions handled in case of incapacity.

**Financial Planning:** Review your financial situation, including assets, debts, and income sources. Consider options like retirement accounts, insurance policies, and long-term care planning to ensure your loved ones are financially secure.

**Communicating Your Wishes:** Openly discuss your legacy plans with your loved ones. Explain your rationale behind specific decisions and ensure they understand your wishes regarding your assets and healthcare. This open communication fosters transparency and avoids any misunderstandings in the future.

**Preserving Family History:** Documenting your family history is a valuable gift you can leave for future generations. This can involve collecting family photos, writing memoirs, recording oral histories, or creating family trees. Sharing your stories and experiences helps future generations connect with their roots and understand their heritage.

**Charitable Giving:** If you are passionate about a particular cause, consider incorporating charitable giving into your legacy plan. Donating to organizations close to your heart allows you to make a positive impact on a cause you care about, even after your lifetime.

Legacy planning is not just about financial security; it is about leaving a lasting impact on your loved ones. Consider incorporating cherished family recipes, letters expressing your love and values, or even digital recordings into your legacy plan. These elements can provide immense sentimental value and serve as a source of comfort and connection for your loved ones long after you are gone.

Remember, legacy planning is not a one-time event. As your circumstances and priorities change throughout life, it is crucial to revisit and update your plans accordingly. Regularly reviewing your will, estate plans, and beneficiary designations ensures your wishes remain accurately reflected and adapt to any changes in your life.

By taking the initiative to create a comprehensive legacy plan, you can ensure your loved ones are taken care of, feel supported, and remember you not only for your financial contributions but also for the love, values, and legacy you leave behind.

## Getting Started with Legacy Planning:

**Gather your financial information:** Organize your financial documents, including bank statements, investment records, and insurance policies.

**Consult with a financial advisor and estate planning attorney:** Seek professional guidance to develop a comprehensive plan tailored to your unique circumstances. They can help you understand legal complexities, navigate various options, and ensure your plan meets your specific needs and goals.

**Talk to your loved ones:** Openly discuss your plans with your family and beneficiaries. Explain your decisions and answer any questions they might have. Encourage them to ask questions and involve them in the planning process as much as they are comfortable.

Regularly review your plans, adapt to changing circumstances, and seek professional guidance when needed. By taking charge of your financial future and expressing your love and values, you can pave the way for a secure, fulfilling retirement and leave a lasting legacy for your loved ones.

DONALD WEST

*"Give a portion to seven, and also to eight; for thou knowest not what evil shall be upon the earth."*

*- Ecclesiastes 11:2 KJV*

# Chapter 8
# Embracing Technology

Let us face it: keeping in touch with loved ones can be tricky, especially as we get older. Maybe you live far away from family, or perhaps getting out and about is not as easy as it used to be. That is where technology comes in! These days, there are all sorts of amazing tools that can help you stay connected with the people who matter most.

This chapter is your guide to using technology to chat, call, and even see your loved ones face-to-face, all from the comfort of your home. Do not worry; even if you are new to gadgets, we will break things down step-by-step.

First things first, a little tech talk. You might need a device to use these tools. Here are your options:

**Cellphones: Your Pocket-Sized Pal:** Cellphones are mini-computers you can carry anywhere! They come in all sizes, so you can find one that fits perfectly in your hand. Big buttons and a bright screen make using them a breeze. Not only can you call and text, but most cell phones also take amazing pictures and videos. Imagine capturing a funny moment with your friends or a beautiful sunset - you can share these memories instantly with the people you love!

**Tablets: Your Entertainment Hub on the Go:** Tablets are kind of like super-sized smartphones. They are bigger and have a wider screen, making them perfect for watching videos, playing games, or video chatting with family and friends. Think of them as entertainment centers you can hold in your hands! They are also great for browsing the internet, so you can look up anything you want to know, from funny cat videos to recipes for your next meal.

**Computers: Powerful Tools for Work and Play:** Computers are the ultimate workhorses. Desktops are the classic kind, the ones you see on desks in offices or schools. They are really powerful and have big screens, which are perfect for getting things done. Laptops are like portable desktops - they are smaller and lighter, so you can easily take them with you wherever you go. Whether you are working on a school project, creating a presentation, or just surfing the web, a computer is a super helpful tool to have around!

Now for the fun part - using these devices to connect! Staying in touch with loved ones is essential, especially as we age. Maybe distance separates you from family, or perhaps your social circle has shrunk.

Whatever the reason, technology offers a solution to combat isolation.

Our trusty phones are a great way to stay connected. Speed dial allows you to program frequently called numbers for easy access. Texting is perfect for quick messages, and many phones offer large buttons and text sizes for easier use. The speakerphone function lets you chat hands-free, which is helpful if holding the phone is difficult.

Feeling like you want to see your loved ones face-to-face? Video chatting is the next best thing! Free apps like Skype, FaceTime, and Google Duo allow you to see and talk with people in real time on your phone, tablet, or computer. These are perfect for catching up with family or having virtual coffee dates with friends. There are also video chat devices with larger screens that connect to your TV, offering an easier navigation option for those with limited vision.

The internet offers a wealth of ways to connect with people who share your interests. Social media platforms like Facebook allow you to connect with friends and family, share photos, and see what is going on in their lives. There are also many senior-focused social media groups where you can connect with people your age who share your hobbies. Online communities and forums exist for practically every interest imaginable. Join the conversation and connect with like-minded people from all over the world!

Trying new things can feel overwhelming, but there are tips to make using technology easier. Start small by focusing on mastering one new tool, like video chatting, before moving on. Do not be afraid to ask for help from grandkids, a friendly neighbor, or even a librarian. Most people are happy to lend a hand! Finally, be patient. Learning new things takes time. Just keep practicing, and you will be a tech whiz in no time!

Remember, the most important thing is to find ways to connect that work for you. Whether it is a daily phone call, a weekly video chat, or joining an online community, there is a tech tool out there to help you stay close to the people you love. So, embrace the possibilities, and get ready to connect!

## Keeping Well with Tech - Health Apps and Wearables for Active Wellness

Taking charge of your health is an important part of living a long and fulfilling life. Today, technology offers a helping hand through a vast array of health apps and wearable devices. These tools can empower you to monitor your well-being, set goals, and make informed choices about your health.

In the world of staying connected to your health, two innovative tools have emerged: health apps and wearables. Health apps are downloadable programs for your phone or tablet that focus on various aspects of well-being. These can track your sleep, diet, exercise, or even blood pressure.

Wearables, on the other hand, are electronic devices you wear, like watches or wristbands. They collect data about your body, such as heart rate, steps taken, or activity levels. Many wearables work seamlessly with health apps, providing a more comprehensive picture of your health by combining the information they gather. This powerful duo empowers you to take charge of your well-being.

Here are some ways health apps and wearables can help you monitor your well-being:

## Health Apps: Your Pocket-Sized Wellness Coach

Health apps come in all shapes and sizes, offering a variety of features to help you stay on top of your health. Here is a glimpse into some popular categories:

**Fitness Trackers:** Have you ever wondered how many steps you take in a day? Health apps can count them! They can also track how far you walk or run, how many calories you burn, and even how many flights of stairs you climb. They do not just measure your activity; they can also help you set goals. Maybe you want to walk for 30 minutes a day or reach a certain number of steps. The app will keep track of your progress and cheer you on!

**Diet and Nutrition Apps:** Do you ever feel lost in the world of nutrition? These apps can be your guide! You can track everything you eat and drink throughout the day, from your morning coffee to your evening snack. The app can then show you how many calories you are consuming and how that compares to your goals. Some apps can even analyze the nutrients in your food, letting you know if you are getting enough vitamins, minerals, and protein.

**Sleep Trackers:** Do you ever toss and turn all night but have no idea how much sleep you are actually getting? These apps can be your sleep detectives! They use the sensors of your phone to track how long you sleep, how often you wake up, and even the different stages of sleep you go through (light sleep, deep sleep, REM sleep). By analyzing your sleep patterns, the app can help you identify any problems you might have, like sleep apnea or trouble staying asleep.

With this, you can develop healthy sleep habits, like going to bed and waking up at consistent times, to improve your sleep quality and feel more rested throughout the day.

### Wearables: Tech You Can Wear!

Wearable devices like smartwatches and fitness trackers take health monitoring a step further. They can be worn comfortably throughout the day and often work seamlessly with health apps to provide a holistic view of your health. Here are some features to look for:

**Heart Rate Monitoring:** Your heart rate is the number of times your heart beats in a minute. It can tell you a lot about your health. A wearable can track your heart rate throughout the day, at rest, and during activity. This can help you identify any potential risks, like an irregular heartbeat.

**Blood Pressure Monitoring:** Not all wearables can do this yet, but some can measure your blood pressure. Blood pressure is the force of blood pushing against the walls of your arteries. High blood pressure, or hypertension, is a major risk factor for heart disease and stroke.

If you have hypertension, a wearable can help you monitor your blood pressure readings and track how well your treatment is working. It can also motivate you to maintain healthy habits that can help lower your blood pressure.

**Sleep Tracking:** Just like sleep tracking apps, wearables can monitor your sleep patterns. They use sensors to track things like your movement, heart rate, and breathing throughout the night.

This can help you understand how well you are sleeping, how long you are in deep sleep and REM sleep (important for memory and learning), and if you are waking up a lot during the night. With this info, you can develop better sleep habits to improve your sleep quality and feel more energized during the day.

**Activity Tracking:** Many wearables are like little fitness trackers on your wrist. They can track things like your steps taken, distance covered while walking or running, calories burned, and even how many minutes you spend actively moving throughout the day.

This data can help you stay motivated to reach your fitness goals. You can set goals for yourself, like taking 10,000 steps a day, and the wearable will track your progress. It can also be a fun way to compete with friends or family in a virtual step challenge!

**Fall Detection:** This is a special feature on some wearables that can be especially helpful for older adults or people at risk of falls. The wearable can detect if you take a sudden fall and send an alert to your emergency contacts or call for help automatically. This can provide peace of mind for you and your loved ones, knowing that help can be called if you have a fall and are unable to get up on your own.

Taking charge of your health is empowering. By using health apps and wearables, you can gain valuable insights into your body, set goals, and make positive changes for a healthier, happier you. So, embrace technology, and let it be your partner on your path to well-being!

## A World of Knowledge at Your Fingertips - Accessing Information and Education Online

As discussed above, the internet has revolutionized how we access information and education. Gone are the days of bulky encyclopedias and limited library hours. Today, with a few clicks or taps, you can explore a vast ocean of knowledge, from the depths of history to the cutting edge of science.

Search engines are your gateway to this vast knowledge. The more specific your keywords or search terms, the more relevant results you will unearth. Most search engines offer advanced search options to refine your results even further. Use quotation marks to find exact phrases and explore Boolean operators (AND, OR, NOT) to narrow down your search. Remember, not all online information is created equal. Be critical of the websites you visit. Look for reputable sources with clear authorship and up-to-date information.

The internet offers a smorgasbord of educational resources, from free online courses to educational websites and articles. Massive Open Online Courses (MOOCs) are a fantastic option. These free or low-cost courses cover a wide range of topics, from history and literature to science and technology. Platforms like Coursera and edX offer courses from prestigious universities around the world.

Many organizations and institutions offer free educational resources on their websites. These may include articles, tutorials, videos, and interactive activities. Local libraries often provide access to online resources like e-books, audiobooks, and digital magazines, all for free with a library card.

The internet provides a wealth of news and information sources. It is important to have a variety of sources for your news to get a well-rounded perspective on current events. With so much information online, it is crucial to be a discerning reader. Check the credibility of websites and fact-check information before sharing it with others. News aggregators can be a convenient way to stay up-to-date on current events. These websites gather news stories from various sources and present them in a centralized location.

## Staying Informed: News Websites and Online Publications

The internet provides a wealth of news and information sources. Here are some things to keep in mind:

**Variety is Key**: Do not rely on a single source for your news. Explore different websites and publications to get a well-rounded perspective on current events.

**Fact-Checking**: With so much information online, it is crucial to be a discerning reader. Check the credibility of websites and fact-check information before sharing it with others.

**News Aggregators**: These websites gather news stories from various sources and present them in a centralized location. This can be a convenient way to stay up-to-date on current events.

While the internet offers a world of knowledge, it is important to be aware of potential risks. Here are some safety tips to keep in mind:

### Unsolicited Emails and Calls:

Be wary of any emails or calls you receive from unknown senders, especially those urging immediate action or offering too-good-to-be-true deals. Legitimate companies would not pressure you into giving away personal information or clicking suspicious links.

Do not open attachments or click on links in emails or messages from unknown senders. These attachments might contain malware, and clicking a link could take you to a fake website designed to steal your information.

Phishing websites often mimic legitimate ones. Before entering any personal information, double-check the website address for typos or unusual spellings. Look for the padlock symbol in the address bar, indicating a secure connection (https).

### Use Strong Passwords:

Strong passwords are your first line of defense against unauthorized access to your online accounts. Do not use dictionary words, birthdays, or personal information in your passwords. Instead, use a combination of uppercase and lowercase letters, numbers, and symbols. The longer and more complex your password, the harder it is to crack.

Avoid using the same password for multiple accounts. If one account gets compromised, hackers can easily access your other accounts with the same password. Remembering multiple complex passwords can be challenging. Consider using a password manager, a secure application that stores and manages your passwords for different accounts. Just remember to create a strong master password for the password manager itself.

## Check the Source:

Before accepting information as fact, consider the source. Is it a reputable news organization, a scientific study, or a personal blog? Look for websites with clear authorship and a history of accurate reporting. Do not rely on a single source of information. Corroborate what you read by checking other credible sources on the same topic. Look for information from multiple perspectives to get a well-rounded understanding.

Be wary of information that relies heavily on emotions or strong opinions rather than facts and evidence. Utilize fact-checking websites to verify information you encounter online. These websites employ professional fact-checkers who research claims and provide reliable information.

The Internet is a powerful aspect of lifelong learning. With a little guidance, you can navigate the online world with confidence and discover a wealth of information and educational resources. So, explore, learn, and enjoy the endless possibilities of online learning!

*"And the Lord God said, It is not good that the man should be alone; I will make him an help meet for him."*

*-Genesis 2:18 KJV*

# Chapter 9
# Taking Charge of Your Life

*"You are your own physician and lifetime planner and investment manager. Jesus is **the** great physician and He authorized you as your planner and gave you the tools you need to take care of yourself, plan for yourself and, to some degree, others that choose to listen and accept your leadership."*

Life can feel like a whirlwind sometimes, especially as we get older. There is so much to keep track of – health, finances, planning for the future. There are times when you cannot help but wonder who is in charge and where to even begin. Well, the good news is, you are! You are the CEO of your own life, and you have to discover the immense power you hold within.

This concept might seem daunting at first. CEO? Is that only supposed to be for bigwigs in fancy suits making million-dollar decisions? Not quite. Think of yourself as the leader of your own life company. You set the direction, manage your resources, and make choices that shape your future. It is an empowering realization – you are not a passive passenger on the journey of life but the driver behind the wheel.

Now, this does not mean you are on your own. Think of it like this: Imagine a grand ocean liner. You are the captain, at the helm, making decisions about the course. But you have a fantastic crew to help you. Your doctor is like the doctor of the ship, ensuring your health. Your financial advisor is the chief navigator, charting the best course for your finances. And most importantly, you have God as your ultimate guide, the captain of all captains. The above-mentioned quote acknowledges Jesus Christ as the Supreme Physician, a source of ultimate healing and guidance. This establishes a foundation of faith, acknowledging that even in moments of struggle or uncertainty, there exists a transcendent source of support and direction.

Let us unpack this quote piece by piece and see how it applies to your life as a senior, a person with a wealth of experience and wisdom.

Being the CEO of your life does not mean you diagnose or treat yourself! But it means you are in charge of your health. You choose healthy foods, get regular checkups, and take any medications as prescribed. You are the one who notices when you do not feel quite right and the one who talks to your doctor about any concerns.

You have lived a long life full of experiences. Now, you get to use that wisdom to plan for the future. This might involve making decisions about your living situation, your finances, or even your healthcare wishes. Do not be afraid to seek advice from professionals like lawyers or financial advisors, but ultimately, the decision should be yours.

Now comes the most important part. It might sound intimidating, but it just means taking care of your finances. You have worked hard for your money, and now you want to make sure it lasts. This could involve talking to a financial advisor to make smart investment choices or simply creating a budget to utilize your money properly.

Even though you are in charge of your health, you are not alone. God is always with you, offering his love, guidance, and strength. Prayer and faith can be a powerful source of comfort and healing. Whether you face a physical ailment or an emotional struggle, turning to God in prayer can bring a deep sense of peace and acceptance.

God has given you everything you need to navigate your life journey. He has given you intelligence, resilience, and experience. You have faced challenges, overcome obstacles, and learned valuable lessons along the way. Draw on that wisdom as you make plans for the future.

He has also given you the gift of free will, the ability to make your own choices. This is a precious gift, and it empowers you to live your life on your terms. Do not let anyone pressure you into decisions that do not feel right. Listen to your inner voice, trust your gut, and make choices that align with your values and desires.

Now, this does not mean Jesus is promising a life free of challenges. Storms will come, both literally and figuratively. But just as a lighthouse helps a captain navigate treacherous waters, Jesus acts as a beacon of hope and strength during difficult times.

Here are some ways Jesus can guide you on your life journey:

**Finding Strength in Faith:** Faith offers a sense of purpose and belonging. Knowing you are part of something bigger than yourself can provide immense comfort and strength, especially in times of hardship. The Bible is full of stories of people who overcame tremendous challenges through their faith in God.

**Inner Peace Through Forgiveness:** Life throws curveballs, and sometimes people hurt us. Jesus emphasized the importance of forgiveness, not for the other person necessarily, but for your own peace of mind. Holding onto anger and resentment is like carrying a heavy burden on your ship. Forgiveness allows you to release that burden and sail on with a lighter heart.

**Love as Your Compass:** The central message that Jesus conveyed was one of love – love for God, love for yourself, and love for your neighbor. This love can be your compass, guiding you toward decisions that bring peace, joy, and connection. When faced with a difficult choice, ask yourself – what would love look like in this situation?

**Gratitude as Fuel:** Taking time to appreciate the good things in life, big or small, can have a profound impact on your well-being. Jesus often expressed gratitude to God the Father. Cultivating an attitude of gratitude can fuel your spirit and help you weather the storms of life.

**Hope for a Brighter Future:** The Bible offers hope for a future beyond this life. Knowing that there may be something more waiting for us can provide comfort and strength, especially as we face the uncertainties of aging and illness. There is no right or wrong way to believe or have faith. However, faith provides a source of strength, comfort, and guidance. Here are some ways to deepen your connection with the great physician:

**Prayer:** Prayer is a powerful way to communicate with God. Talk to him about your worries, hopes, and dreams. Thank him for the blessings in your life.

**Scripture:** The Bible is filled with wisdom and guidance. Reading scripture, even a few verses a day, can offer comfort, inspiration, and a deeper understanding of your faith.

**Fellowship:** Connecting with a faith community can be incredibly rewarding. Sharing your journey with others can offer support and encouragement.

Then comes the next part of the quote. As a senior, you have a wealth of wisdom to share. You can be a guiding light for younger generations, offering your advice and support if they want it.

So, dear reader, embrace your role as the captain of your ship. Take charge of your health, your plans, and your finances. With God as your guide and your own inner wisdom as your compass, you can navigate the rest of your life journey with confidence and peace.

# Activity to Spark Your Wisdom and Leadership

### Mentor a Younger Person

Think outside the box! Volunteer at a local school and mentor students in a subject you are passionate about. Offer to coach a youth sports team, sharing your knowledge and fostering a love for the game. Become a pen pal with a child overseas, exchanging letters and sharing cultural experiences.

### Write a Memoir or Legacy Letter:

Make it a multimedia project! Scan old photos and create a scrapbook alongside your written memoir. Record yourself telling stories and compile them into an audio memoir. Use online platforms to create a website or blog dedicated to your life story.

### Volunteer Your Time and Skills:

Find a cause you care about and turn it into an adventure! Volunteer at an animal shelter and walk dogs or cuddle cats. Help plant trees at a local park and contribute to the green spaces in your community. Offer your computer skills at a senior center and help others navigate the digital world.

### Join a Senior Center or Social Group:

Do not just join any group; find one that ignites your passions! Look for social groups dedicated to hobbies you enjoy, like book clubs, gardening clubs, or photography clubs. Participate in senior center activities that pique your interest, from line dancing classes to watercolor painting workshops.

Taking charge of your life is a journey, not a destination. Be patient with yourself and celebrate your progress. Do not be afraid to ask for help. There are many resources available to assist you with your health, finances, and planning for the future. Most importantly, embrace this new chapter in your life. Remember that There is a higher power, a great physician, guiding you and offering strength and love along the way.

## Strengthening Your Shield: The Power of Vaccinations for Seniors

Besides spiritual and mental wellness, keeping up with physical health and well-being is equally significant. As we age, our bodies undergo many changes, including a weakening immune system. This leaves us more susceptible to serious infections and complications that can significantly impact our health and well-being. However, there is a powerful weapon at hand: the shield of vaccinations and immunizations. These vital injections offer invaluable protection for seniors, acting as a barrier against harmful diseases and safeguarding their golden years.

Our immune system is tasked with defending us against invading pathogens like bacteria and viruses. However, with age, this defense mechanism becomes less efficient. The production of white blood cells decreases, our immune response weakens, and our ability to remember past infections diminishes. This decline in immunity makes seniors more vulnerable to a range of potentially life-threatening diseases.

Vaccinations and immunizations work by mimicking the natural process of infection without causing the actual illness. This triggers the immune system to create defenses, or antibodies, specific to the targeted disease. These antibodies remain in our bodies, ready to swiftly fight off future encounters with the pathogen. This pre-armed response significantly reduces the risk of developing the disease or experiencing severe complications if infected.

Getting vaccinated not only protects the individual but also contributes to the immunity of the community. This is similar to creating a protective bubble around those who cannot get vaccinated, such as people with certain medical conditions. Seniors play a vital role in maintaining this shield of protection for the whole community.

Vaccination guidelines may change over time, and new vaccines may become available. It is crucial for seniors to stay informed and regularly discuss their vaccination status with their healthcare providers. This ensures they have the most up-to-date protection against emerging health threats.

Some seniors may be hesitant about vaccinations due to concerns or misinformation. Open communication with healthcare professionals can address these concerns and provide accurate information. Understanding the benefits of vaccinations is key to embracing them as powerful tools for staying healthy.

So, vaccinations and immunizations are the superheroes in the battle against infectious diseases. Seniors can enhance their well-being by staying updated on recommended vaccines, creating a robust defense system that keeps them resilient and contributes to the overall health of the community.

### Key Vaccinations for Seniors:

Here are several crucial vaccinations recommended for seniors:

**Influenza:** The annual flu vaccine protects against seasonal influenza strains, significantly reducing the risk of severe illness, hospitalization, and even death.

**Pneumococcal:** This vaccine safeguards against pneumococcal bacteria responsible for pneumonia, meningitis, and other serious infections.

**Tetanus, diphtheria, and pertussis (Tdap):** This booster shot protects against tetanus, diphtheria, and whooping cough, diseases that can be particularly dangerous for older adults.

**COVID-19:** Getting vaccinated and boosted against COVID-19 remains crucial for seniors due to their increased risk of severe illness and complications.

**Hepatitis B:** Protects against a liver infection.

**Zoster (shingles) booster:** This can offer further protection against recurring shingles.

## What to Expect During a Check-up:

### 1. Physical Examination:

Your doctor will perform a physical examination, checking various aspects like blood pressure, heart rate, and general well-being.

### 2. Blood Tests and Screenings:

Blood tests and screenings may be conducted to check cholesterol levels, blood sugar, and other important markers for various health conditions.

### 3. Discussing Lifestyle Factors:

Your doctor will likely discuss your lifestyle, including diet, exercise, and sleep patterns. This allows for personalized advice on maintaining a healthy lifestyle.

### 4. Reviewing Medications:

The doctor will review any medications you are taking, ensuring they are effective and not causing any unwanted side effects.

This is your time to discuss any health concerns or symptoms you may be experiencing. Open communication with your doctor is key to receiving the best care possible.

### 5. The Role of Authority:

Many people accept whomever they determine as the "authority" as not just knowing what is best but that they could not suggest something that was not the absolute best for them. This might not be true, so everyone should recognize that they are the person really in charge of their well-being.

Certainly, listen to the authority giving advice, recommendations, or direction, but it is your responsibility to take care of yourself, not theirs. If you know that a medicine or a procedure has been questioned or not thoroughly tested, reconsider jumping into the unproven since you are your own commander-in-chief. It hinges on you. If you have a good friend or loved one, get their opinion before taking the dive.

Remember, you are your own doctor (advisor, manager, dietitian, dentist).

Remember, regular check-ups are a vital part of maintaining good health as we age. By staying proactive and scheduling routine medical examinations, seniors can enjoy a better quality of life and ensure that they are taking the necessary steps to stay healthy and happy. Do not forget your health is an investment in your future well-being!

*"Thou shalt rise up before the hoary head, and honor the face of the old man, and fear thy God: I am the Lord."*

*- Leviticus 19:32 KJV*

# Chapter 10
# Aging Like a Champion

We have finally reached the end of our journey together, learning all sorts of ways to stay healthy as we get older. This whole book was not about trying to be young forever; it was about feeling fantastic at every age, like a total champion!

Throughout this book, we have discussed strategies to keep your mind sharp, your body strong, and your spirit vibrant. Remember, healthy aging is not about chasing after your youth. It is about making the most of each stage in life and finding ways to thrive, no matter your age.

Let us think back to all the cool tricks that we have learned. We talked about yummy and healthy foods that give your body the energy it needs to do awesome things. Just like a car needs good gas, you need good food to keep going! Remember, eating lots of fruits, veggies, and whole grains makes you feel like a winner. We discovered delicious ways to cook these healthy foods, turning mealtimes into celebrations.

We also discovered the power of moving your body. Even a little bit of exercise each day, like a walk around the block or some stretches, can make a big difference. Exercise is like giving your body a high five

— it gets stronger and has more energy to do the things you love. Maybe you have discovered a new exercise you enjoy, like dancing in your living room or swimming in the pool. Remember, finding ways to move that you have fun with makes it easier to stick with it.

Spending time with loved ones, laughing, and sharing stories keeps your spirit bright and your heart happy. Taking care of your mental health is just as important as taking care of your body. Maybe you have some aches and pains that come with getting older. That is okay! There are ways to manage them and stay active. Talk to your doctor and find out what exercises are right for you. There are also lots of tools and techniques to help you manage any pain you might have.

But being healthy is not just about your body. Keeping your mind sharp is important, too! We talked about trying new hobbies, learning new things, and having fun chats with friends. The more you use your brain, the sharper it stays, just like a muscle you keep exercising. Maybe you picked up a new craft, started reading more books, or even decided to learn a new language. Remember, challenging your mind keeps you feeling young and keeps the world interesting.

Most importantly, we talked about the magic of a positive attitude. The way you think about things can really affect how you feel about getting older. Remember to focus on the good stuff, like spending time with loved ones, learning new things, and all the amazing experiences you have collected over the years. Be thankful for what you have, and never give up on your dreams. A positive attitude is sunshine for your soul – it makes everything seem brighter and happier.

Getting older is actually an amazing thing. As the years go by, you collect all sorts of wisdom and experiences, like cool trophies on a shelf. These are the stories you share with others, the things you teach them, making you a wise and awesome person. You have built strong relationships, learned valuable lessons, and seen so much of the world. Embrace the wisdom that comes with age, and share it with those around you.

Never stop growing and learning! There is always something new to discover, no matter your age. Be open to new experiences, embrace challenges, and keep your curiosity alive. Remember that even small changes in your life can make a big difference in your journey. By taking care of yourself, you can stay active and independent for many years to come.

By staying healthy and active, you can keep exploring this wonderful world for a long time. Imagine yourself at seventy, full of life and stories.

With a little bit of effort and a positive outlook, you can reach your eighties and even beyond. The world is waiting to be explored, so keep that adventurous spirit alive! This is your journey, and every twist and turn is a part of the amazing story of your life.

As you reach the milestone of your nineties, may "Aging Gracefully" be your trusted companion on this remarkable journey. By adopting a holistic and comprehensive approach to health, maintaining a positive mindset, and embracing the opportunities that each day brings, you can truly thrive in your later years. Here is to a life rich in experiences, wisdom, and the joy that comes with aging gracefully.

So, make the most of your golden years. Spend time with the people you love, try new things that make you happy, and just enjoy life. By following the tips in this book and keeping a smile on your face, you can keep feeling like a champion every single day. You are not defined by your age but by how awesome you make your life. Go out there and be the best you can be every step of the way! You have got this, champion!

# Activity: Design Your Champion Aging Plan!

Congrats on finishing the book and learning all these amazing tips for healthy aging! Now, it is time to put them into action and design your very own Champion Aging Plan.

### Here is What You Can Do:

### 1. Fuel Your Body:

* Make a list of your favorite healthy foods from what you learned in the book.

* Pick 2-3 new fruits or vegetables you would like to try this week.

* Plan a champion breakfast, lunch, and dinner that incorporates these healthy choices.

### 2. Move Your Body:

* Think about what exercises you enjoyed in the book (walking, dancing, swimming).

* Choose an activity you will do for at least 15 minutes and 3 times this week.

* Put it on your calendar and set a reminder!

### 3. Sharpen Your Mind:

\* Recall a hobby you wanted to try or a new skill you wanted to learn.

\* Dedicate 30 minutes this week to exploring it (reading about it, watching a tutorial, taking a practice session).

### 4. Brighten Your Spirit:

\* Call a friend or family member you have not spoken to in a while and schedule a catch-up call or visit.

\* Write down 3 things you are grateful for today.

### 5. Reflect and Recharge:

\* Think about how you are feeling overall.

\* If you are feeling stressed, write down your worries and brainstorm some solutions.

\* Make sure you are getting enough sleep each night to feel your best.

Remember, this is just a starting point. As you go through your week, keep adding new healthy habits and activities to your Champion Aging Plan. You have got this!

*"And we know that for those who love God all things work together for good, for those who are called according to his purpose."*

*-Romans 8:28-30 KJV*

## About the Author

Donald West was born on October 10, 1932, at home 319 South East 43rd St, in Oklahoma City, where he lived until the family moved to Arkansas in 1949 because his father, an oil derrick safety engineer, received a job transfer. He attended Shields Heights Elementary, Capitol Hill Junior High, and Capitol Hill High School till the eleventh grade when the family moved, and he had to attend Little Rock High School for his senior year. Little Rock High School was chosen as the most beautiful high school in the United States and was built in 1927. Don West was into journalism and was assigned as head of the photography division as a senior, graduating in 1950.

On his seventeenth birthday, while still in high school, he joined the United States Naval Reserves, with his father witnessing his swearing in. Don went to boot camp in Great Lakes, Illinois, and a Navy cruise out of New Orleans for Cuba and Haiti. Upon returning, he learned that his family had moved back to Oklahoma City without him, and the family residence was empty, awaiting the new owners. In Oklahoma, towards the end of his junior year at Capitol Hill High School, Donald West had applied to attend Oklahoma University, but those plans were shelved when the family moved to Arkansas.

On enrollment day, he and his best friend since they were four years old, went to O.U. to enroll in the fall of 1950. Both friends chose the Army Reserve Officer Training Corps and joined the Pershing Rifles Society, named after WWI General John J. Pershing. Donald became their President in his senior year, as well as the captain of the Army ROTC Rifle Competitive Team. Rather than accept an Army Second Lieutenant Commission, he became interested in flying and chose the U. S. Navy Flight Training in Pensacola.

Following the multi-engine training in Hutchison, Kansas, and earning the Navy Wings of Gold, he returned to Pensacola, Florida, as a primary flight instructor in the formidable SNJ, an advanced trainer from WWII, and used by many nations in combat using guns, rockets, and bombs. Although Ensign West did his share of single engine aviation instructor duty. His interests included gliders and private cross-country in single engine with family. Most of his Navy patrol flying was over the sea along the coasts of antagonistic countries, reporting on shipping commercial fishing all over cold, fierce seas as a Lieutenant and around the Vietnam area as a Lieutenant Commander but flying as an Attaché Duty in Africa as a Commander.

Following the Attaché tour, he attended George Washington

University, acquiring a master's degree in 1972 and CBN University in 1980-1982 for Television Camera and acquiring a second master's degree at Regent University in Electronic Journalism in 2002.

Commander West had planned to live long enough to see his grandchildren graduate from high school, but that has recently become most difficult because, at first, his 55-year-old son considers all the surfers he taught surfing to as his offspring, his legacy, but then he married and at 63, has a seven-year-old son and a five-year-old daughter.

Doing the math now, it looks like the author must reach 103 to attend the high school graduation of his granddaughter.

Made in the USA
Middletown, DE
25 June 2024